Speech Acoustics and Perception

ARTHUR BOOTHROYD

pro·ed

8700 Shoal Creek Boulevard
Austin, Texas 78758

The PRO-ED
studies in
communicative disorders

Series editor
HARVEY HALPERN

Library of Congress Cataloging in Publication Data

Boothroyd, Arthur
  Speech acoustics and perception.

  (The PRO-ED studies in communicative disorders)
Bibliography: p.
  1. Speech perception. 2. Speech—Physiological
aspects. I. Title. II. Series.
BF463.S64B66 1986   414   86-3236
ISBN 0-89079-079-5

pro·ed

8700 Shoal Creek Boulevard
Austin, Texas 78758

10 9 8 7 6 5 4 3 2   91 92 93 94 95

Contents

PART FOUR
The Sense of Hearing

PART FIVE
Auditory Speech Perception

Preface

The communication of ideas via spoken language is an activity that is unique to human beings. The process involves first the formulation of the ideas to be communicated and then the representation of those ideas by combinations of symbols. The symbols we call *words* and the combinations of words we call *sentences*. The complete set of possible words, together with the rules for combining them into sentences, constitute a *language*. When language is expressed in its spoken form, the words and sentences are represented by movements of the speech mechanism. These movements, in turn, produce sound patterns that become the evidence on which a listener must base decisions about the words, sentences, and ideas they represent.

This process is exceedingly complex and only partially understood. Yet every normal child learns to produce and to perceive the sound patterns of spoken language without formal instruction and at a very young age. So spontaneous is the acquisition and use of spoken language skills that most people are unaware of the special nature of this activity, or of its complexity.

The purpose of this text is to provide an introduction to that part of the process dealing with the generation and perception of the sound patterns of language. It is written for the beginning student in communication sciences or communication disorders and for students or workers in allied professions. No advanced knowledge of mathematics or science is assumed. The text begins with a review of the nature and structure of sound patterns in general and moves on to the mechanisms by which we generate the special sound patterns of speech. A description of the specific sound patterns of English follows, and the text ends with a discussion of hearing and the way it is used to interpret the sound patterns of language.

Because of the introductory nature of this material, and in the interests of readability, references to the scientific literature have been avoided in the text itself. Instead, there is a bibliography that will lead the interested reader to more advanced treatments of the topics covered here.

I am grateful to my colleague Professor Katherine Harris for valuable comments on earlier drafts of this material, and to the many students who have served as catalysts for thought.

PART ONE

Sound

Language, as an activity, is not restricted to any particular form or medium. Think, for example, of written language, sign language, Morse code, and Braille, and you will realize the variety of ways in which the human capacity for language can be expressed. Spoken language, however, is intended to be heard and is therefore specifically dependent on sound for its transmission between a talker and a listener. For a brief moment in time the symbols of language exist as sound patterns in the air between two people. It is therefore with sound that our discussion will begin.

The Nature of Sound

We use the word *sound* to describe movement patterns in the air that are capable of stimulating the human sense of hearing. Sound is produced by events involving the rapid movement of an object. Some examples are the snapping of a twig, the turbulent flow of water when it encounters an obstacle, and the vibrations of a guitar string after it is plucked. The movements of the object cause corresponding movements of the surrounding layers of air. Air is an elastic medium that resists compression and expansion. Movements of one layer of air therefore cause movements of the adjacent layer, which cause movements in the next layer, and so on. The patterns of movement therefore travel away from their source in the form of waves, much as ripples spread across the surface of a pond when a stone is thrown in the middle.

As sound travels from its source, the patterns of movement in the air replicate the patterns of movement in the originating event. In this way, sounds carry evidence about the events that caused them. The use of our sense of hearing to detect and interpret sound patterns is one of the ways by which we learn about events occurring in the world around us.

Sound Patterns

Pure Tones

The patterns of movement that constitute sound are usually very complicated. All sound patterns, however, are made from the same basic building blocks, called *pure tones*. When a pure tone is present, the air particles vibrate back and forth about their normal position with a movement pattern that is smooth and repetitive. The movement patterns in a pure tone are like those of a swinging pendulum, only much faster. A pure tone is completely described by just two quantities, frequency and amplitude.

The *frequency* of a pure tone is the number of repetitions of the movement pattern occurring in 1 second. We refer to each repetition as a single cycle and can therefore express frequency in cycles per second (cps or c/s). It is currently standard practice, however, to replace cycles per second with hertz (Hz), which means exactly the same thing. When we refer to a pure tone of frequency 1000 Hz, we mean that the air particles are vibrating back and forth 1,000 times per second.

The human sense of hearing is capable of responding to pure tones whose frequencies are in the range 20 Hz to 20,000 Hz. Vibrations whose frequencies are less than 20 Hz are referred to as "infrasound." Vibrations whose frequencies are higher than 20,000 Hz are referred to as "ultrasound."

The *amplitude* of a pure tone is the size of the repetitive movements (i.e., the distance traveled by the air particles as they vibrate back and forth). We do not, however, usually measure sound amplitude in terms of distance. Instead, we use the *decibel* (dB) scale. On the decibel scale, each increase of 10 dB represents a 10-fold multiplication of sound energy. If, for example, we let 0 dB represent the amplitude of a reference sound, then at 10 dB the energy is 10 times that of the reference sound, at 20 dB the energy is 100 times that of the reference sound (i.e., 10 × 10, or two multiplications by 10). At 30 dB the energy is 1,000 times that of the reference sound (i.e., three multiplications by 10), and so on. The main justification for this approach is that the human sense of hearing responds to equal multiplications of sound energy as roughly equal additions of loudness.

The range of human hearing, from the quietest audible sound to the loudest tolerable sound, is approximately 100 dB. This means that the loudest sound we can tolerate is some 10 billion times as strong as the quietest sound we can detect. If we let 0 dB represent the amplitude of the quietest sound we can hear, then sounds that are too weak to be heard will have negative decibel values and sounds with amplitudes in excess of 100 dB will be too loud for comfort.

Pure tones are the building blocks of more complex sound patterns. A complete description of the frequencies and amplitudes of a sound's constituent pure tones is known as its *spectrum*. The spectrum is to sound what the list of ingredients is to a recipe. Each pure tone is an ingredient. The identity of that ingredient is specified by its frequency, while the amount required is given by its amplitude. The details of a sound's spectrum provide a listener with important clues about the nature of the event that caused the sound.

Complex Sounds

Sounds whose spectra consist of two or more pure tones are referred to as *complex sounds*. They are of two basic types, complex tones and random noise.

Complex tones are generated by such things as a violin, a trumpet, and the human vocal cords. What these sources have in common is that they involve repetitive movements. In this respect, they are like pure tones. The difference is that the movement patterns are more complicated.

Because the movement patterns repeat themselves, there is a definite time period for each cycle. We therefore describe the movement patterns of complex tones as *periodic* (i.e., with period). The frequency with which the patterns repeat themselves is known as the *fundamental frequency* of the complex tone.

When we examine the spectrum of a complex tone, we find an orderly relationship among the frequencies of the constituent pure tones. Each is a whole-number multiple of the fundamental frequency. For example, in a complex tone whose fundamental frequency is 300 Hz, we find that the constituent pure tones have frequencies of 300 Hz, 600 Hz, 900 Hz, 1200 Hz, and so on.

Note that these frequencies are 1 × 300 Hz, 2 × 300 Hz, 3 × 300 Hz, 4 × 300 Hz, and so on. We refer to the constituent tones of a complex tone as *harmonics*, numbering them in sequence. Thus, in the example just given, the frequency of the first harmonic is 300 Hz, the frequency of the second harmonic is 600 Hz, and so on.

In *random noise*, the patterns of movement do not repeat themselves. Examples are the sounds made by a snapping twig, by the turbulent flow of water, by a snare drum, and by air as it escapes through a narrow opening. Because the vibration patterns are not repetitive, no time period can be observed and the patterns may therefore be described as *aperiodic* (i.e., without period).

In the spectrum of a random noise we can observe no orderly relationships among the frequencies of the constituent tones. Instead, we find energy spread broadly across wide ranges of frequency, as if there were thousands of harmonics packed tightly together.

Another way in which complex sounds can differ from one another is in the patterns of change of amplitude over time. Some sounds begin and end gradually. Others begin and end abruptly. Some last for a considerable time, while others are transient, ending almost as soon as they begin. The pattern of change of amplitude over time is known as the *time/intensity envelope*, and, like the spectrum, is an important source of information about the nature of the event from which the sound originates.

The spectrum of a sound can also change over time, slowly or quickly, smoothly or abruptly. These changes, too, carry information about the event that caused the sound. The sound patterns of human speech include both complex tones and random noise, and involve frequent, rapid changes of both intensity and spectrum over time. They are very complex, complex sounds.

Behavior of Sound in Air

Speed

The movement patterns that constitute sound travel through the air at a speed of about 1,000 feet per second. (Note that it is the patterns that are moving, not the air. The phenomenon can be compared to an electric billboard in which individual lights turn on and off to produce a moving pattern. It is the patterns that move, not the lights.) Because of the finite speed of sound, there is a delay between the occurrence of an event and the arrival of the resulting sound patterns at our ears. At a baseball game, for example, there can be a noticeable delay between seeing and hearing the ball strike the bat (roughly 0.5 seconds if you are 500 feet from the batter), and in a thunderstorm we can estimate the distance by timing the delay between a lightning flash and the associated thunderclap (about 1 mile for every 5 seconds). At short range, the delays are much smaller. If, for example, we are conversing with someone who is 10 feet away, there will be a delay of about 1/100th of a second between the time when we see the movements of speech and the time when we hear the sounds they produce. And if someone speaks to us from our right side, the right ear will receive the sound patterns about 1/1000th of a second before the left ear.

Change of Amplitude with Distance

As sound moves away from its source, the sound energy spreads over an ever-increasing area and the concentration of sound therefore diminishes. If the source of sound is very small, if the sound is radiated equally in all directions, and if there are no reflecting surfaces, we can show that the amplitude falls by 6 dB for every doubling of distance. Thus, if you are standing 5 feet from me and receiving my speech at a level of 60 dB (with reference to the quietest sound you can hear), you could theoretically double your distance 10 times before I would become inaudible. This would take you to a distance of 5,000 feet, or roughly 1 mile. Because sound can travel over considerable distances and still remain audible, hearing is an excellent early-warning system for animals.

Effect of Obstacles

When sound waves strike a large smooth surface, they are reflected in the same way that light is reflected from a sheet of glass. This reflection gives rise to the phenomenon of the echo.

When sound is produced in a room, the reflections from the walls, ceiling, and floor are so numerous and so rapid that we cannot distinguish individual echoes. Instead, there is a general persistence of sound that we refer to as *reverberation*. Designers of lecture rooms, theaters, and concert halls go to great lengths to adjust the reflectivity of the inside surfaces in order to obtain the correct amount of reverberation.

Although sound behaves like light in some ways there is one very important difference between the two forms of energy. Light always travels in straight lines, but sound travels around corners. If, for example, we put an obstacle in the path of light, we block it completely, casting a shadow. If, however, we put an obstacle in the path of sound, some of the sound waves that miss the obstacle change direction and "fill in" the shadow. The fact that sound travels around corners makes it possible for animals to hear events that cannot be seen, providing yet another survival advantage. This behavior of sound is also important to speech, since it permits us to hear movements such as those of the vocal cords, even though they are out of sight.

Resonance

Because of a particular combination of weight and elasticity, most mechanical systems have one or more frequencies at which they will vibrate naturally. That is, if these systems are disturbed and then left alone, they will vibrate at some natural frequency as they return to their original condition. Examples are a stretched string, which vibrates at a natural frequency when plucked; a gong, which vibrates at a natural frequency when struck; and child on a swing, which vibrates at a natural frequency when given a push.

If we try to force a mechanical system to vibrate, we find that it is relatively easy as long as we match the stimulating frequency to a natural frequency. At any other frequency we require a lot of energy, and the resulting amplitude is very small. (Just try pushing a child's swing at a rate other than its natural one.) At a natural frequency, however, we require only a little energy to produce large amplitudes of vibration.

Resonance is the name used to refer to the production of large amplitudes of vibration in a system by stimulating it at a natural frequency. The classical example is of a wine glass—which, by singing at a natural frequency, we can shatter by using resonance to produce large amplitudes of vibration.

When air is enclosed in a cavity, it exhibits natural frequencies of vibration. These arise from a particular combination of the elasticity, or springiness, of a trapped volume of air, and the weight, or inertia, of a moving volume of air. If a pure tone enters the cavity, its behavior will depend on its frequency. At frequencies other than a natural frequency, the air in the enclosure will vibrate with low amplitude. If, however, the frequency of the pure tone equals a natural frequency of the air in the cavity, resonance will occur and the amplitude of vibration will be large.

You will recall that a complex sound contains many pure tones. When a complex sound enters an enclosed space, only those constituent pure tones that match a natural frequency will produce large amplitudes of vibration. In this way, the phenomenon of resonance can modify the spectrum of a complex sound, causing prominent spectral peaks (i.e., frequency regions in the spectrum in which the constituent pure tones are of high amplitude) at natural frequencies of vibration. This process is of crucial importance to the production of human speech, where resonance occurs in the cavities of the nose and mouth.

It is sometimes easier to understand the resonant behavior of trapped volumes of air by using a mechanical analogy. Consider, for example, a container

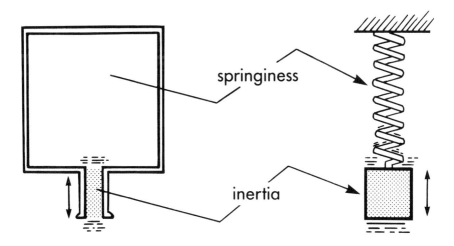

Figure 1. The air in a bottle behaves like a spring in that it resists compression or expansion. The air in the neck has inertia in that it requires a force to start it moving, or to stop it if it is already moving. The behavior of the air in the neck of the bottle is like that of a weight on the end of a light spring. If disturbed, they both bounce up and down at a natural frequency. Increasing the size of the bottle lowers the natural frequency, as does lengthening and narrowing the neck. This system is often referred to as a Helmholtz resonator, in memory of the scientist who first studied it in detail.

such as a fat bottle with a short, narrow neck (see Figure 1). The air in the bottle acts as a spring, pushing against the air in the neck if it tries to move into the bottle and pulling it back if it tries to escape. The air in the neck, though very light, has a certain amount of inertia – that is, it requires a little effort to make it move or to stop it if it is already moving. The air in the bottle therefore behaves very much like a spring with a weight on the end. If you pull on the weight and let go, it will bounce up and down at its natural frequency. Similarly, if you disturb the air in the neck of the bottle, it will vibrate back and forth at its natural frequency.

The natural frequency of the air in the bottle depends on two things: the volume of the cavity and the size of the neck. A low natural frequency occurs when the cavity is large and the neck is long and narrow. A high natural frequency occurs when the cavity is small and the neck is short and wide.

If, in the last example, we give the cavity and the neck the same diameter, we produce a tube of constant cross section (see Figure 2). At first sight it seems as though we have removed the weight from the spring. In reality, however, just as a real spring has weight of its own, so the air in the tube has inertia of its own. In the first example, the inertia was concentrated in the neck

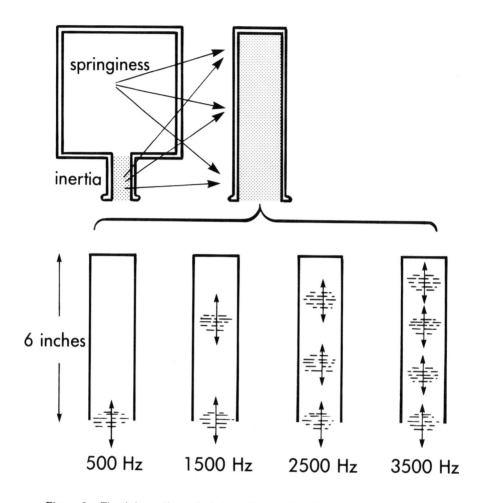

Figure 2.   The air in a uniform tube behaves like a spring with weight distributed evenly along its length. Such a system can be made to vibrate in several ways, each with a different natural frequency. The values of the frequencies are related to each other, however, each being an odd-numbered multiple of the lowest one.

of the bottle. Now it is distributed uniformly along the length of the tube. It is as though we had taken the weight from the end of the spring and distributed it uniformly along the spring. A system such as this has not just one natural frequency but several. In a uniform tube of the same length as that of an adult male vocal tract (roughly 6 inches), for example, the natural frequencies are

500 Hz, 1500 Hz, 2500 Hz, 3500 Hz, and so on. Note that each of these frequencies is an odd-numbered multiple of the first.

To understand why the air in a uniform tube has more than one natural frequency, we must return to the concept of sound as waves that travel through the air at a speed of about 1,000 feet per second. In a pure tone, the "peaks" of these waves follow each other at a rate equal to the frequency of the tone. At 1000 Hz, for example, a peak passes by every 1/1000th of a second, and between each peak there is a "trough."

When the tone enters a tube, it is reflected back and forth between the two ends. It is easy to understand how the sound is reflected from the closed end, but at first sight we would expect it simply to escape when it reaches the open end. In fact, it is the discontinuity that reflects the sound, and there is a discontinuity at both the closed and the open ends. There is, however, a difference in the reflections at the two ends. At a closed end, a peak in the wave is reflected as a peak, and a trough is reflected as a trough. At an open end, a peak is reflected as a trough, and a trough is reflected as a peak.

As the sound is reflected back and forth between the ends of the tube, there are certain frequencies at which all the peaks and all the troughs in the multiple reflections are in step with each other, adding together to produce large amplitudes of vibration. These are the natural frequencies of vibration.

Recall that a peak leaving the closed end travels down the tube and is reflected from the open end as a trough. If it arrives back in one half of a cycle, it will be in step with the next trough of the wave. If it arrives back in three half cycles, it will be in step with the next trough but one. If it arrives back in five half cycles, it will be in step with the next trough but two, and so on. Since sound travels at 1,000 feet per second, it will take 1/1000th of a second to travel to the end of a 6-inch tube and back. The natural frequencies of the tube therefore have values such that 1/1000th of a second equals one half cycle, three half cycles, five half cycles, and so on. A little calculation shows that the periods for these frequencies are 1/500th of a second, 1/1500th of a second, 1/2500th of a second, and so on. Recall that frequency is the number of cycles occurring in 1 second. Now it can be seen why the natural frequencies of a 6-inch tube, open at one end and closed at the other, are 500 Hz, 1500 Hz, 2500 Hz, and so on, in odd-numbered multiples of 500 Hz.

Measuring Sound

Several instruments have been developed for the measurement, examination, or analysis of sound patterns. I shall describe only three: the sound level meter, the oscilloscope, and the sound spectrograph.

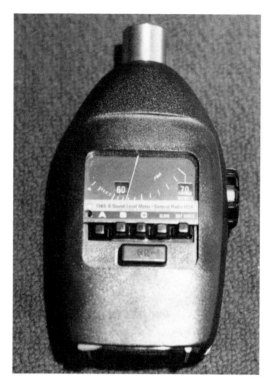

Figure 3. Sound level meters are used for measuring the amplitude of sound vibrations. They are calibrated to read amplitude in decibels, the value of 0 dB being assigned to a sound with a precisely specified amplitude.

Sound Level Meter

The sound level meter contains a microphone to convert sound patterns to electrical signals, an electronic amplifier to magnify the electrical signals, and a meter, calibrated in decibels, to measure them. The main purpose of the sound level meter is to measure the amplitude of sound patterns. When measuring complex sounds, various methods are used to "average" the amplitudes of the constituent pure tones. Figure 3 shows a typical sound level meter in use.

Oscilloscope

The oscilloscope is a general-purpose instrument designed for displaying electrical signals. It can be used for examining the vibration patterns of sound by

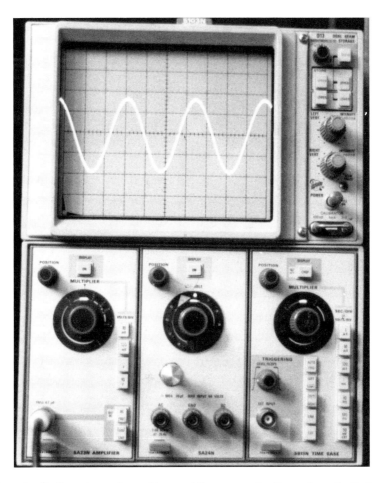

Figure 4. Oscillographs can be used to reveal the movement patterns of sound with the help of a microphone that converts movement patterns into electrical signals. The resulting pictures are called oscillograms.

first converting these patterns into electrical signals with a microphone. The resulting visual patterns, called *oscillograms*, show time horizontally and air movements vertically. Figure 4 shows an oscilloscope in use, and Figure 5 shows typical oscillograms for a pure tone, a complex tone, a random noise, and a short sample of speech. Note the smooth repetitive pattern of the pure tone, the complicated but still repetitive pattern of the complex tone, the complicated, nonrepetitive pattern of the random noise, and the presence of both complex tones and random noise in the sample of speech.

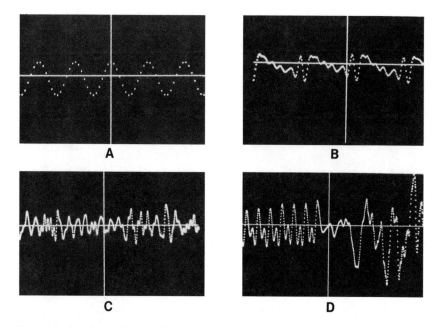

Figure 5. Sample oscillograms. A, a pure tone; B, a complex tone; C, a random noise, and D, a short sample of speech.

Sound Spectrograph

The sound spectrograph is designed for the analysis of rapidly changing sound patterns such as those of speech. It first records a short sample of sound, either magnetically or in a computer memory. This sample is then played repeatedly while the machine looks for energy at each frequency, starting with the lowest and ending with the highest. A drum rotates in time with the repeated replays, and if sound energy is found, a dark trace is left on a sheet of paper attached to the drum. The result is a *spectrogram* (sometimes known as a "voice print"), which shows time horizontally, frequency vertically, and amplitude as the degree of blackness. Figure 6 shows a sound spectrograph in use, and Figure 7 shows typical spectrograms for a pure tone, a complex tone, a random noise, and a short sample of speech. Note the single frequency in the spectrum of the pure tone, the regularly spaced harmonics in the spectrum of the complex tone, the absence of a regular harmonic structure in the spectrum of the random noise, and the mixture of complex tones and random noise in the spectrum of the speech sample.

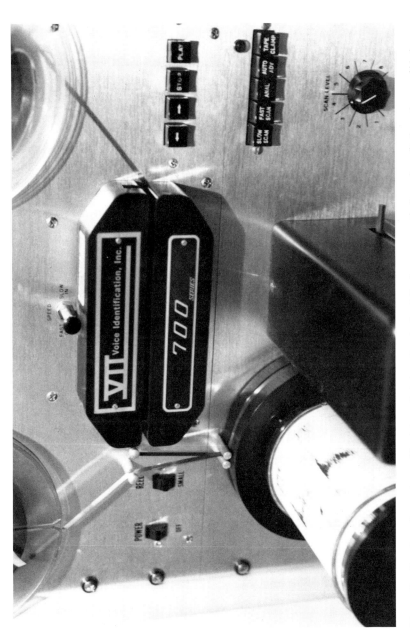

Figure 6. Sound spectrographs provide pictures that show time horizontally, frequency vertically, and amplitude as degree of blackness. These pictures are known as spectrograms.

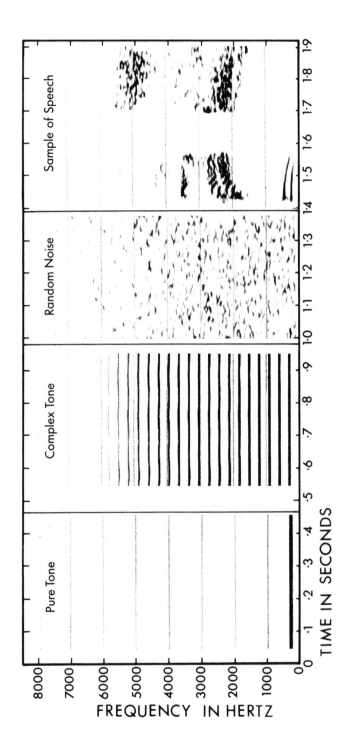

Figure 7. These sample spectrograms illustrate that (a) the spectrum of a pure tone contains only a single frequency, (b) the spectrum of a complex tone contains many tones whose frequencies are harmonically related, (c) the spectrum of a random noise contains energy that is spread across a broad range of frequencies, and (d) the spectrum of speech contains both complex tones and random noise, with many changes of amplitude and spectrum in a relatively short time.

PART TWO

Speech

As part of their evolutionary development, human beings have capitalized on the properties and behavior of sound as a medium for communication. The thoughts to be communicated by one individual are coded in the form of language patterns (i.e., words and sentences), which are, in turn, coded in the form of movement patterns. The movement patterns generate patterns of sound that are detected by another individual who uses them to deduce the language patterns they represent, and hence the original thoughts. We use the term *speech* to refer to three aspects of this communication process: the overall process of representing language by sound, the motor behaviors that produce the sounds, and the resulting patterns of sound themselves. The intended use of the term is usually obvious from context. If there is a possibility of confusion, this can be avoided by referring to the *speech process*, *speech movements*, and *speech sounds*, respectively.

15

Speech Mechanism

The sounds of speech are produced by structures whose functions were originally limited to breathing and eating. These structures include the lungs, the larynx, the mouth, and the nasal passages, together with their associated muscles and the neural systems that control them.

A simplified cross-sectional diagram of the speech mechanism is provided in Figure 8. This mechanism has six active sections: the lungs, larynx, velum, jaw, tongue, and lips. The *lungs*, after inhalation, contain a reservoir of air that, under the combined influence of the elasticity of the rib cage and the muscles of the abdomen and chest, becomes an outward flow of air. This outward air flow is the basis for speech sound production. The *larynx* contains the vocal folds (also known as the vocal cords), which can be brought together to interrupt the flow of air from the lungs. The *velum* is a soft, muscular flap at the back of the palate that can be lowered to allow the flow of air and sound into the nasal cavity, or raised to prevent it. The *jaw* can be raised or lowered, thus changing the size of the oral cavity. The *tongue*, which is the most mobile part of the mechanism, can be moved upwards, downwards, backwards, and forwards, thus changing both the shape and size of the oral cavity and, if necessary, interrupting the air flow. The final section is the *lips*, which are also mobile and can be used to change the shape and size of the opening of the oral cavity and, if necessary, to interrupt the air flow. Speech production requires rapid, precise, and coordinated control of these six sections of the speech mechanism.

Process of Speech Sound Production

There are three stages in the process of speech sound production. First, a flow of air is created. Second, this air flow is made to generate sound by placing obstructions in its path. Third, the spectrum of the resulting sound is modified by resonance within the cavities of the nose and mouth.

One way of looking at this process is in terms of sound sources and sound filters. Interruption of the flow of air produces a *sound source*. The result is a complex sound, either a complex tone or a random noise, whose spectrum contains many pure tones. In order to reach the outside air, this sound must pass through one or more cavities. Those tones within the sound spectrum whose frequencies coincide with a natural frequency of the air in the cavities cause resonance—that is, they produce large amplitudes of vibration and are therefore transmitted efficiently to the surrounding air. Other tones produce only small amplitudes of vibration and are therefore transmitted inefficiently to the sur-

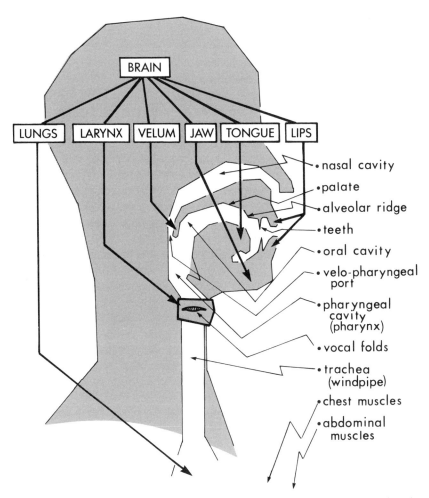

Figure 8. A simplified cross-sectional diagram of the speech mechanism. There are six active sections. After inhalation, the lungs contain a reservoir of air that can be made to flow steadily outwards by the combined action of the muscles of the chest and abdomen. The larynx contains the vocal cords that can be used to interfere with the outward air flow to produce the sound of the voice. The velum is essentially a valve that can be raised, thus preventing air and sound from entering the nasal cavity, or lowered, thus allowing air and sound to enter the nasal cavity through the velopharyngeal port. The jaw can be raised or lowered to change the size of the oral cavity. The tongue can be moved about to change the shape and size of the oral cavity and, if necessary, it can produce a complete or partial blockage by contacting the upper teeth, the alveolar ridge, the palate, or the velum. The lips can also be used to change the shape and size of the oral cavity, and, if necessary, the lower lip can produce a complete or partial blockage by contacting the upper lip or the upper teeth. Speech production requires rapid, precise, and coordinated control of these six active sections of the speech mechanism.

rounding air. The cavities of the mouth and nose act like a filter, allowing some frequencies to pass easily while holding back others, just as a coffee filter allows the coffee to pass through but holds back the coffee grounds. This is the *source-filter* description of the speech production process (see Figure 9).

It was pointed out earlier that sound patterns carry evidence about the nature of the events that produced them. From the foregoing it will be seen that the sounds of speech carry two kinds of evidence. The first is evidence about the source of sound—that is, how it was produced. The second is evidence about the acoustical properties of the cavities, or filter, through which the sound has passed. The sound systems of spoken language employ variations in the characteristics of both the sound sources and the filter in order to convey information. Because the people who listen to speech are also experienced producers of speech, they know how to interpret the evidence carried by speech sounds in terms of the speech movements that caused them.

In spoken English, all speech sounds are produced from the outward flow of air from the lungs (i.e., during exhalation). We use three different types of sound source: voicing, frication, and stop-plosion. The spectra of the resulting sounds are modified by resonance in two cavities, the mouth and the nose. In the following sections, the three sound sources and the two resonant cavities will be discussed in more detail.

Sound Sources

Voicing

Voice production occurs only in the *larynx*, a complex structure at the opening of the windpipe. This structure consists of numerous cartileges, internal muscles, and external muscles. Within the larynx are the *vocal folds*, two partly muscular shelves between which the air must pass as it leaves the windpipe. The space between the vocal folds is known as the *glottis*. This space can be made smaller by bringing the vocal folds closer together, or larger by moving them farther apart. If the vocal folds are brought together during exhalation, the escaping air causes them to vibrate, alternately opening and closing the glottis. The air is thus released in brief, repetitive bursts, generating a complex tone, called *voicing*. The same effect can be produced by allowing the air to escape through the stretched neck of an inflated balloon. The sound pattern of voicing has a periodic vibration pattern and a harmonic spectrum.

The *fundamental frequency* of voicing is the frequency at which the vocal folds vibrate. The average values of fundamental frequency are approximately

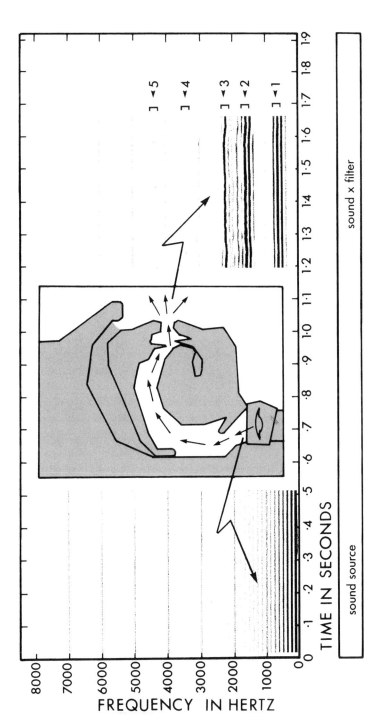

Figure 9. Speech production involves a sound source and a filter. A complex sound (either a complex tone or a random noise) is generated within the mechanism. In order to reach the outside air, this sound must pass through one or more cavities. Those pure tones in the source spectrum that coincide with a natural frequency of the air in the cavities will cause resonance, thus acquiring high amplitude and being transmitted to the surrounding air very efficiently. The spectrum of the emerging sound therefore contains prominent peaks at the natural frequencies of the cavity. Five such peaks can be seen in the spectrogram shown here.

100 Hz, 200 Hz, and 250 Hz in men, women, and children, respectively, the differences being due to differences in the size and weight of the vocal folds.

During the production of speech, we introduce changes of the fundamental frequency of voicing, above and below its average value. These changes, which are produced by tightening or relaxing the vocal folds, are heard as the melody, or *intonation*, of speech. In men, the fundamental frequency rises and falls between a low value of about 70 Hz and a high value of about 200 Hz. In women, the range is roughly 140 Hz to 400 Hz, and in children it is roughly 180 Hz to 500 Hz.

Figure 10 shows spectrograms of a speech sample whose sole source was voicing. The first spectrogram was produced with a narrow analyzing filter that reveals the individual harmonics of the voice spectrum. It will be seen that the fundamental frequency rises and falls during this utterance. As it does so, the frequencies of all the pure tones in the spectrum rise and fall with the fundamental frequency. The second spectrogram was produced with a wider analyzing filter that obscures the fine details of the spectrum but shows the individual openings of the vocal folds as fine vertical striations. It will be seen that, as the fundamental frequency rises, the openings of the vocal folds follow each other more rapidly. This second type of spectrogram is the one most widely used in examining the sounds of speech. Because voicing is a complex tone, it has a harmonic spectrum in which the component frequencies are whole-number multiples of the fundamental frequency. The amplitudes of the harmonics, before they are modified by resonance, fall at a rate of approximately 12 dB for every doubling of frequency. If, for example, the amplitude of the first harmonic were to have an amplitude of 72 dB, the second harmonic would have an amplitude of 60 dB, the fourth harmonic an amplitude of 48 dB, the eighth harmonic an amplitude of 36 dB, and so on. This fact is not evident in the spectrograms of Figure 10 since the sound had already been modified by passing through the oral cavity before being recorded by the spectrograph.

There are marked individual variations of the average fundamental frequency, the range of fundamental frequency, and the spectrum of voicing. These variations contribute to the qualities that make it possible for us to recognize an individual from the sound of his or her voice.

Frication

Frication is produced by forcing air through a narrow opening at a high enough rate to cause turbulent flow. The resulting sound is a random noise. The vibration patterns are aperiodic, and the spectrum covers a wide range of frequencies, with a predominance of the higher-frequency components. Figure 11 shows the spectrogram of a speech sound in which frication is the sole source.

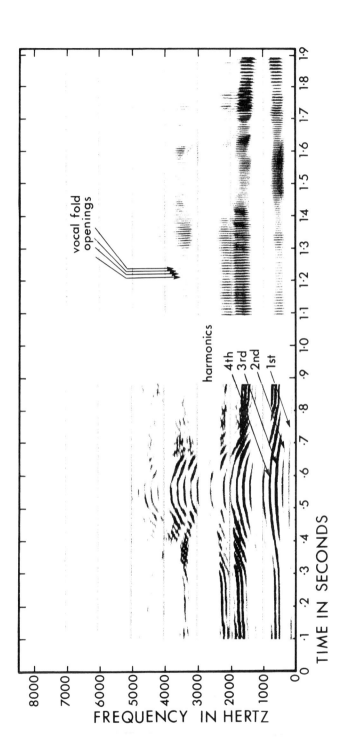

Figure 10. These two spectrograms are of a speech sound pattern whose only sound source was voicing. During this utterance, the fundamental frequency was made to rise and then fall. Two types of spectrograms are shown. In the first, a very narrow analyzing filter was used so that the details of the harmonic structure of the voicing could be seen. Note that all the harmonics rise and fall with the fundamental. In the second spectrogram, a wider analyzing filter was used. This obscures the details of harmonic structure but provides improved detail in the time domain, showing each opening of the vocal cords as a fine vertical stripe. Note that the openings follow each other more rapidly as the fundamental frequency rises. The second type of spectrogram is the one most frequently used in speech science research and will be used for most of the illustrations in the remainder of this text.

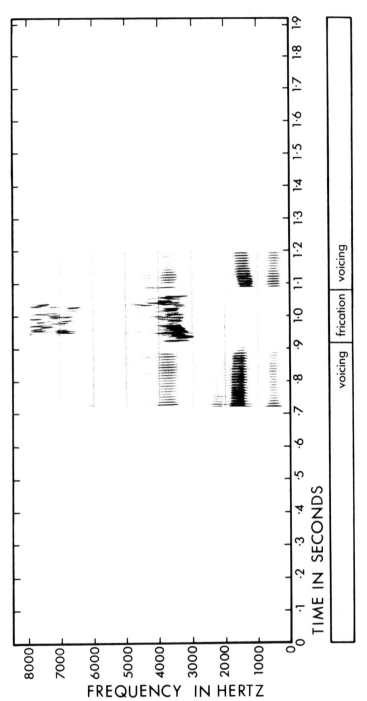

Figure 11. In this spectrogram we see, between two voiced sounds, a sound pattern whose sole sound source is frication. Note the irregularity (i.e., randomness) of the fine vertical striations, the broad spread of frequencies, and the predominance of high frequencies.

Unlike voicing, which is produced only in the larynx, frication can be produced anywhere in the vocal tract. All that is needed is the creation of a narrow gap through which the air must flow. We refer to the place at which this gap is created as the *place of articulation*. The different places of articulation, named according to the surfaces between which the gap is created, are as follows:

1. *Bilabial* — between the lower lip and the upper lip

2. *Labiodental* — between the lower lip and the upper teeth

3. *Linguadental* — between the tongue and the upper teeth

4. *Alveolar* — between the tongue and the alveolar ridge (the gum ridge behind the upper teeth)

5. *Palatal* — between the tongue and the hard palate

6. *Velar* — between the tongue and the soft palate, or velum

7. *Glottal* — between partially closed vocal folds

Note that the efficient production of frication anywhere but at the glottis requires a substantial flow of air through the mouth. This will not happen unless the velum is raised to prevent air from escaping into the nasal cavity. This is just one of many examples of the coordination that is required among different sections of the speech mechanism.

Stop-Plosion

Stop-plosion is produced by a complete stoppage of air flow, followed by release of the air pressure that builds up during the stoppage. The sound pattern of stop-plosion consists of a period of silence during the "stop" portion, lasting about 1/10th of a second, followed by a sudden burst of random noise (i.e., an "explosion") as the air flow resumes, lasting about 1/20th of a second. The spectrum of the random noise is similar to that of frication produced at the same place. Its amplitude envelope, however, is very different. The amplitude rises from zero to a very high value at the moment of release of air pressure and then returns to zero very rapidly as the opening through which the air is escaping becomes wider. Figure 12 shows the spectrogram of a speech sound whose sole source is stop-plosion.

Stop-plosion can be produced anywhere in the vocal tract where there can be a complete interruption of air flow. The spaces between the teeth make it difficult to produce labiodental or linguadental stops. This leaves five places of articulation: bilabial, alveolar, palatal, velar, and glottal. The raising of the velum,

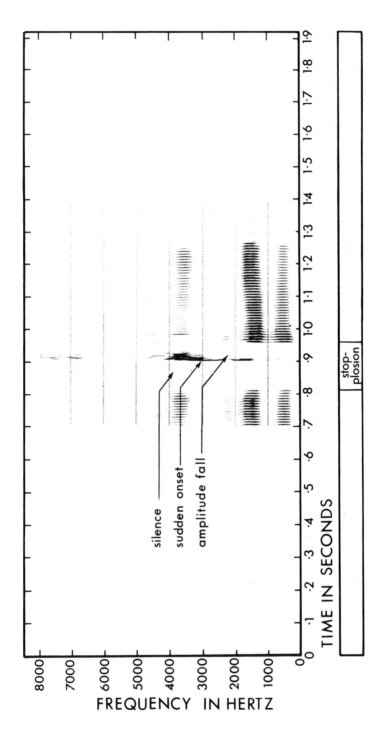

Figure 12. In this spectrogram we see, between two voiced sounds, a sound pattern whose sole sound source is stop-plosion. Note the period of silence during the interruption of air flow, the sudden onset of random noise as the built-up air pressure is released, and the rapid reduction of amplitude of the random noise as the opening through which air escapes becomes larger.

in order to prevent air from escaping through the nose, is as important for stop-plosion as it is for frication.

The three types of sound source just described can be used separately or together, thus giving us the following seven different sound-source variations from which a sound system can be developed:

1. voicing alone

2. frication alone

3. stop-plosion alone

4. voicing plus frication

5. voicing plus stop-plosion

6. frication plus stop-plosion

7. voicing plus frication plus stop-plosion

Resonant Cavities

The Oral Cavity

The oral cavity is an irregularly shaped tube that, in men, measures about 17 cm (just over 6 inches) from larynx to lips. In women and children it is some-what shorter. As explained earlier, the air in this tube has several modes of vibration (i.e., ways of vibrating), each with a different natural frequency. Each mode of vibration is referred to as a *formant*. The formants are identified by number, starting with the one having the lowest frequency. That is, the mode of vibration with the lowest natural frequency is the first formant (F1), the one with the next-lowest frequency is the second formant (F2), and so on. The formants produce prominent peaks in the spectrum of the emerging speech sound. These peaks appear as dark bands on wide-band speech spectrograms, as seen in Figures 10, 11, and 12. Note that although, strictly speaking, these bands show the spectral peaks that are produced by formants, it is common practice to refer to the spectral peaks themselves, and even to the dark bands on the spectrogram, as formants.

In men, the *average frequency* of F1 is about 500 Hz, but, by changing the shape and size of the oral cavity, this frequency can be varied from around 300 Hz to around 900 Hz (i.e., over a range of about 3:1). The average frequency of F2 is about 1500 Hz, but it too can be varied, from around 900 Hz to around 2700 Hz (also a range of about 3:1). Subsequent formants have average frequencies that go up in steps of about 1000 Hz (2500 Hz, 3500 Hz, etc.). These frequencies also change with changes in the shape and size of the oral cavity, but not as much as do the frequencies of F1 and F2. The changes of formant frequencies that occur in running speech are illustrated in the spectrogram of Figure 13. Since the vocal tracts of women and children are shorter than those of men, the average frequencies of the formants are consequently higher.

To understand how changes in the shape and size of the oral cavity modify the frequencies of the first two formants, we must return to the earlier discussion of resonance and think of the oral cavity as a uniform tube, closed at the larynx and open at the lips. The natural frequencies of vibration of each tube, if 17 cm long, are 500 Hz, 1500 Hz, 2500 Hz, and so on, in odd-numbered multiples of 500 Hz. The closest approximation to this condition with a real vocal tract is obtained by sustaining the vowel in the word *head* (see Figure 14).

If we now raise the tongue toward the palate and at the same time reduce the size of the lip opening, we narrow the tube both in the middle and at the opening. In effect we have produced two cavities, a back cavity and a front cavity. The mechanical analogy is of two weights connected by two springs. Going from the uniform tube to the two-cavity condition is analogous to taking the weight that is uniformly distributed in a spring and concentrating it in two "lumps," one in the middle and one at the end (see Figure 15).

The first formant may be thought of as due to interaction between the springiness of the back cavity and the combined weight of the air in the two tubes. The value of the first-formant frequency falls as the two tubes are narrowed (i.e., as the tongue or jaw is raised and the lip opening made smaller). It also falls as the back cavity is made larger (i.e., as the tongue is moved forward). The second formant may be thought of as due to the interaction between the springiness of the front cavity and the weight of the air in the lip opening. The value of the second-formant frequency falls as the front tube is narrowed (i.e., as the lip opening is narrowed and extended). It also falls as the front cavity is made larger (i.e., as the tongue is moved back or the jaw is dropped).

The two-cavity model just presented is an oversimplified description that fails to take into account the fact that the air in the cavities has some weight and the air in the tubes has some springiness. Nevertheless, it helps us to understand the basic articulatory correlates of the frequencies of the first two formants.

It will be seen from the foregoing that any change in jaw position, tongue height, tongue place (front-back), or lip opening will affect the frequencies of both F1 and F2. Nevertheless, by coordinating the activities of the jaw, tongue,

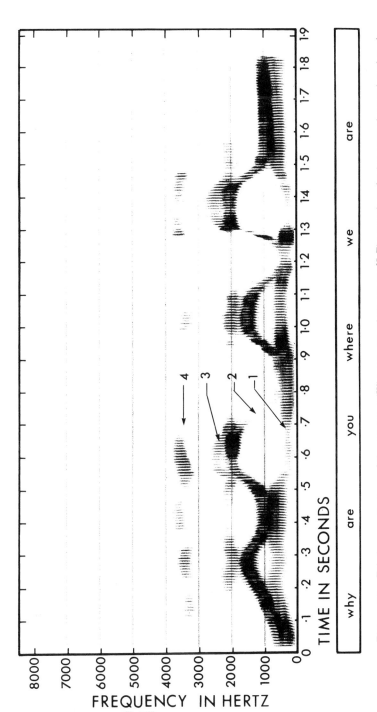

Figure 13. This is a spectrogram of the utterance "Why are you where we are?" The mouth cavity has several natural modes of vibration, or formants. When a complex sound, such as voicing, enters the mouth cavity, resonance occurs at the frequencies of the formants, producing peaks in the spectrum of the sound emerging from the lips. These peaks appear as dark bands on the spectrogram. As the jaw, tongue, and lips move, the size and shape of the oral cavity changes, thus changing the formant frequencies.

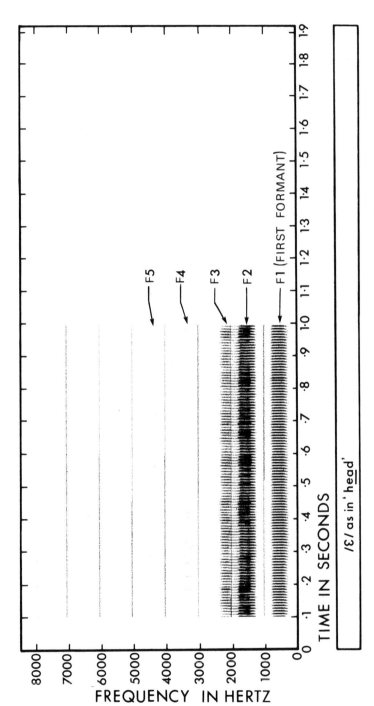

Figure 14. When producing the vowel in the word *head*, the vocal tract comes close to resembling a tube of uniform cross-section. In the adult male, this tube has a length of approximately 6 inches and the formant frequencies are close to the predicted average values of 500 Hz, 1000 Hz, 1500 Hz, and so on, in odd-numbered multiples of 500 Hz.

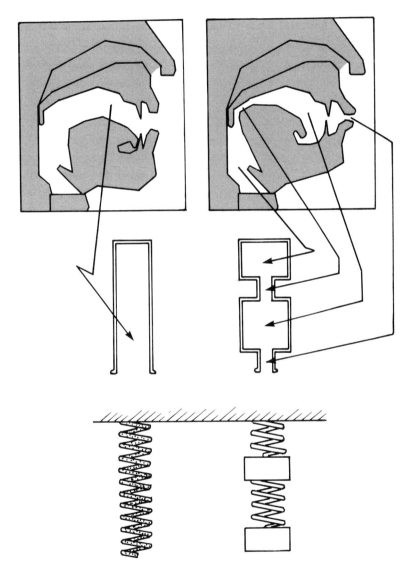

Figure 15. As we raise the tongue and narrow the lips, the mouth cavity ceases to resemble a tube of uniform cross-section and more closely resembles two cavities connected by a tube, a second tube connecting them to the outside air. The mechanical analogy is of two weights and two springs. The frequencies of the formants are now determined by the amounts of "springiness" of the air in the two cavities and the "weight" (more correctly, the inertia) of the air in the two tubes. Note that this is an oversimplified description that ignores the springiness of the air in the tubes and the inertia of the air in the cavities.

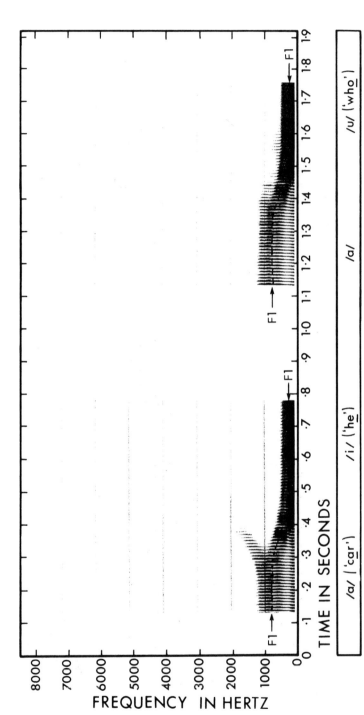

Figure 16. The frequency of the first formant depends mainly on the size of the back cavity and the length and width of the connecting tubes. These dimensions depend, in turn, on the positions and configurations of the tongue, the jaw, and the lips. Although all three work in concert, the most direct relationship is seen between first formant frequency and the height of the tongue. In the spectrograms shown here, the tongue is moved from its lowest position (as in the vowel in *car*) (a) to its highest position at the front of the mouth (as in the vowel in *he*) and (b) to its highest position at the back of the mouth (as in the vowel in *who*). In both cases, the frequency of the first formant falls from its highest value to its lowest value (in these samples from 800 Hz to 300 Hz).

and lips we can attain virtually independent control of these two formants. Under these conditions, the frequency of F1 is highly correlated with the *height* of the tongue. This relationship is illustrated in Figure 16, which shows the effect of changing from an open cavity to a relatively closed one (i.e., changing from the position for the vowel in *hod* to that for the vowels in *who'd* or *heed*).

Similarly, the frequency of F2 is highly correlated with the *place* of the highest part of the tongue in relation to the front of the mouth. This relationship is illustrated in Figure 17, which shows the effect of changing from a front placement to a back placement (i.e., changing from the position for the vowel in *heed* to that for the vowel in *who'd*).

In the illustrations used so far, the effect of resonance in the oral cavity was considered only for the situation in which the sound source is voicing. Resonance also occurs when the sound source is frication or stop-plosion, as will be seen in the spectrogram of Figure 18.

By lowering the velum, we open the velopharyngeal port and allow resonance to occur in the nasal cavity. We can think of this, like the oral cavity, as a uniform tube that is closed at one end and open at the other. It therefore has a series of formants whose frequencies are roughly odd-numbered multiples of the lowest frequency. Since the length of the tube is greater than that of the oral cavity, the formant frequencies are correspondingly lower (see Figure 19).

Unlike the oral cavity, the nasal cavity has a relatively fixed shape and size. The formant frequencies cannot, therefore, be changed very much. We can, however, introduce small modifications by closing off the oral cavity at different places to create a side cavity of variable size, as illustrated in Figure 20.

Note that we have three possible configurations of the oral and nasal cavities: (1) oral cavity alone (velum raised), (2) nasal cavity with a side tube (velum lowered and oral cavity blocked), and (3) oral and nasal cavities together (velum lowered and oral cavity left open).

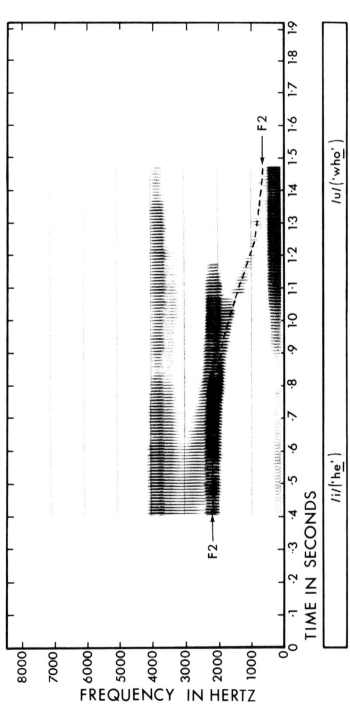

Figure 17. The frequency of the second formant depends mainly on the size of the front cavity and the length and width of the lip opening. These dimensions depend, in turn, on the positions and configurations of the tongue, the jaw, and the lips. Although all three work in concert, the most direct relationship is seen between second formant frequency and the position of the highest part of the tongue in relation to the front and back of the mouth. In the spectrogram shown here, the tongue is moved from its most frontal position (as in the vowel in *he*) to its most rearward position (as in the vowel in *who*). In the process the frequency of the second formant falls from its highest value to its lowest value (in this sample from 2200 Hz to 700 Hz).

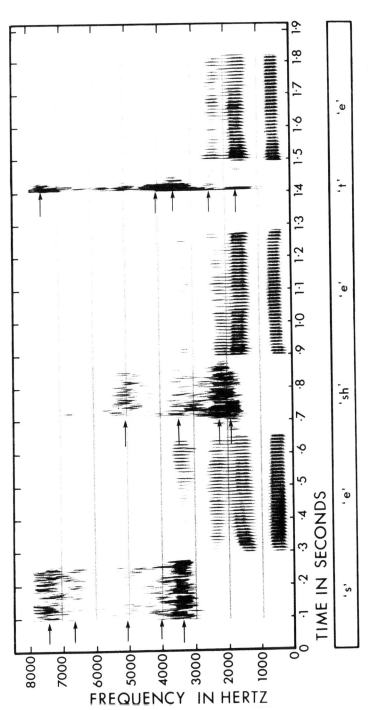

Figure 18. Although evidence of formants is seen most clearly in sounds whose sole source is *voicing*, resonance also plays an important role in sounds whose sole source is either frication or stop-plosion. Note the prominent bands of energy in the spectra of these samples of the sounds *s*, *sh*, *t*, shown here between voiced sounds. (The vowel that separates these sounds is the vowel in the word *head*).

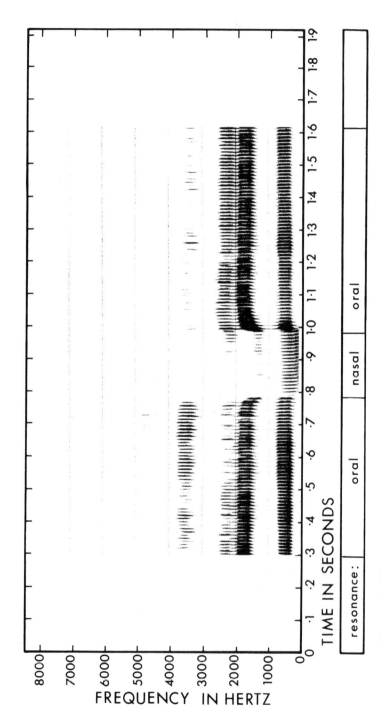

Figure 19. When the only resonant cavity is that of the nose, resonance occurs at the frequencies of the nasal formants. These formants are lower in frequency that those of the oral cavity, and the amplitude of the sound emerging from the nose is rather low, as seen in this spectrogram of an *m* sound, produced between two vowels.

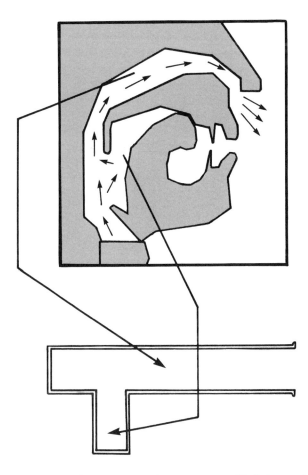

Figure 20. In order to restrict resonance to the nose, we must block the mouth cavity. This creates a side cavity whose size depends on the position of the blockage. As we change the size of this side cavity we produce subtle changes in the frequencies of the nasal formants.

PART THREE

The Sound Patterns of Language

The speech mechanism described in the previous section is capable of generating an enormous range of discriminable sound patterns. The speakers of any given language, however, use only a limited selection of these patterns for transmitting messages. *Phonetics* is the study of the sound patterns of languages. *Phonology* is the study of the ways in which these sound patterns are organized in order to convey information.

Phonemes

The sound patterns of a given language can be arranged in classes, or groups, according to their role in determining word meaning. Each class is called a *phoneme*. Two sound patterns belong to the same phoneme if they can be interchanged without altering word meaning, whereas two sound patterns belong to different phonemes if the substitution of one for the other results in a change of word meaning. For example, the first sound pattern in the word *spoon* (i.e., the *s*) involves a different mouth shape and a different spectrum from the *s* in the word *sea*. And yet if we took the *s* from the word *sea* and replaced it with the *s* from the word *spoon*, we would not have changed the meaning of the word. These two versions of *s* therefore belong to the same phoneme class. In contrast, if we took the *s* from the word *see* and replaced it with the *t* from the word *too*, we would produce a word with a new meaning, namely *tee*. These two sounds therefore belong to different phoneme classes.

When we want to express, in writing, the name of the phoneme to which a speech sound pattern belongs, we usually place the appropriate symbol between slashes. For example, in the previous paragraph we were discussing the phonemes /s/ and /t/. The symbols generally used to represent phonemes have been agreed upon internationally. The complete set is known as the International Phonetic Alphabet (IPA). Many of the symbols are identical to those used in written English, but some represent different sound patterns. In this text I shall accompany phonetic symbols with key words in order to avoid confusion.

The phonemes of English can be divided into two major groups, the vowels and the consonants.

Vowels

The usual sound source for vowels is voicing. (I say "usual" because it is possible to produce whispered vowels in which the sound source is glottal frication.) The sole resonator is the oral cavity. There are some 17 vowels in English. They fall into three groups: long vowels, short vowels, and diphthongs.

Long Vowels

The *long vowels*, as the name suggests, tend to occupy more time than short vowels. There are roughly six long vowels in English, differentiated at the articulatory level by the shape of the oral cavity and at the acoustical level by the frequencies of the formants, especially F1 and F2. When reading the following descriptions, you should also refer to the spectrograms and formant plots shown in Figure 21.

1. /a/ (*hod*) is produced with the tongue in a mid position, neither front nor back, and as low as it can go. With the oral cavity in this configuration, the first formant is at its highest value and the second formant is at its lowest value.

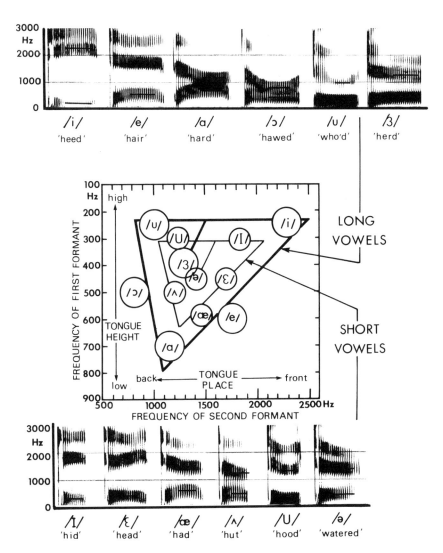

Figure 21. On a plot of the frequency of F1 versus the frequency of F2, the six long vowels are roughly enclosed by a triangle with /a/, /u/, and /i/ at the corners. The vowel triangle for the short vowels is somewhat smaller, reflecting the more restricted range of articulatory movements. Note that these data are taken from single examples of one adult male speaker. There is a wide range of variation in vowel production within and among speakers.

2. /i/ (*heed*) is produced with the tongue high and forward. At the same time the lips are spread and retracted. With the oral cavity in this configuration, the first formant has its lowest value and the second formant its highest value.

3. /u/ (*who'd*) is produced with the tongue high and back. At the same time the lips are rounded and protruded. With the oral cavity in this configuration, both the first and second formants have their lowest values.

On a plot of tongue height versus tongue place (front/back), or on a plot of first-formant frequency against second-formant frequency, the three vowels /a/, /i/, and /u/ are close to the points of a triangle that encloses all of the vowels. For this reason they are referred to as the *point vowels*. Between these point vowels we find three other long vowels:

4. /e/ (*hairdo*) falls along one side of the vowel triangle defined by the point vowels. It is roughly halfway between /i/ and /a/.

5. /ɔ/ (*hawed*) also falls along one side of the vowel triangle, between /a/ and /u/.

6. /ɜ/ (*heard*) is a neutral vowel, neither high nor low, front nor back. It falls roughly in the center of the vowel triangle.

Short Vowels

For each of the long vowels we can define a *short vowel* produced with similar articulatory configuration. Each short vowel typically occupies less time than its long counterpart. Corresponding with the three point vowels /a/, /u/, and /i/ are the following short vowels:

1. /ae/ (*had*)

2. /U/ (*hood*)

3. /I/ (*hid*)

It will be seen from Figure 21 that the vowel triangle defined by these three vowels is smaller than that defined by the three point vowels. Within this triangle we find three other short vowels:

4. /ɛ/ (*head*)

5. /ʌ/ (*hut*)

6. /ə/ (*watered*)

Diphthongs

The *diphthongs* are essentially "double vowels." They begin as mid or low long vowels and end as high short vowels. Their main characteristic is the movement of the articulators, which produces corresponding changes of formant frequencies. This is illustrated in the spectrograms of Figure 22. The diphthongs of English are:

1. /eI/ (*hayed*), which begins as /e/ and ends as /I/.

2. /aI/ (*hide*), which begins as /a/ and ends as /I/.

3. /ɔI/ (*hoyed*), which begins as /ɔ/ and ends as /İ/.

4. /aU/ (*how'd*), which begins as /a/ and ends as /U/.

5. /ɔU/ (*hoed*), which begins as /ɔ/ and ends as /U/.

The 6 long vowels, 6 short vowels, and 5 diphthongs give us a total of 17 vowels. The articulatory classification of these vowels is summarized in Table 1.

There is considerable variability in the vowel systems of persons from different countries or different regions of the same country, even though they may speak the same language. The foregoing analysis and the examples provided in Figure 21 are from a single speaker and are by no means representative of "Standard American English." Note also that the exact articulatory configuration, and therefore acoustic pattern, of a given vowel phoneme varies considerably within the speech of a given speaker, depending on phonetic context and stress.

Consonants

The consonants generally occupy less time than do vowels. They also tend to be weaker, to contain more high frequencies (above 1000 Hz), and to involve more rapid movements of the articulators. There are some 25 consonants in English. They fall into five categories: vowellike consonants, nasals, fricatives, stop-plosives, and affricates. These will be discussed in turn.

Vowellike Consonants

Vowellike consonants are similar to vowels in that the sole source is voicing and the sole resonator is the oral cavity. They tend, however, to be weak and short-lived and to involve rapid movements of the articulators. Spectrograms of vowellike consonants show formants that depend on the shape and size of the

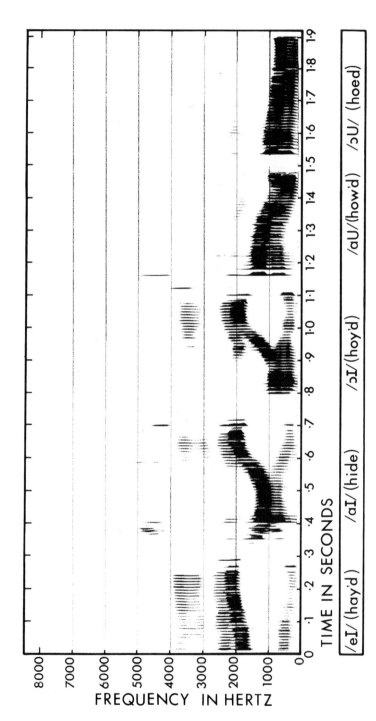

Figure 22. The English diphthongs are characterized by movement from one vowel configuration to another. These movements appear as changes of formant frequency in the vowel spectra.

TABLE 1
Classification of Long and Short Vowels by Tongue Height and Place

			Tongue Place				
			Back	Mid		Front	
	High	Long	/u/			/i/	
Tongue		Short		/U/			/I/
Height							
	Mid	Long	/ɔ/	/3/		/e/	
		Short		/ʌ/	/ə/		/ɛ/
	Low	Long		/a/			
		Short		/ae/			

Note: The five diphthongs begin as low or mid long vowels (/ɔ/, /a/, or /e/) and end as high short vowels (/U/ or /I/).

oral cavity. These formants change rapidly, however, as the articulators move. There are four vowellike consonants in English:

1. /w/ (*will*) is like the vowel /u/ in that it is produced with rounded and protruded lips. The lips immediately move, however, into the position for the vowel that follows.

2. /j/ (*you*) is like the vowel /i/ in that it is produced with a high front tongue position. The tongue immediately moves, however, into the position for the vowel that follows. Because the articulators "glide" into position to anticipate the vowel that follows, the consonants /w/ and /j/ are referred to as *glides*. Their primary acoustical characteristic is the rapid change of formant frequencies as the articulators change position (see Figure 23).

3. /r/ (*read*) is like the vowel /3/ in that it is produced with the tongue in a neutral position.

4. /l/ (*life*) is an unusual sound in that the tip of the tongue makes contact with the alveolar ridge, but the sides are dropped to permit air and sound flow to continue. Because of this feature, the sound /l/ is also referred to as a *lateral*. A key acoustical feature of /l/ is the sudden change of formant frequencies as the tongue touches and then leaves the palate (see Figure 23).

Nasals

In *nasals*, the sound source is voicing, and the resonator is the nasal cavity with the mouth as a closed side cavity. To produce the nasals, the velum must be

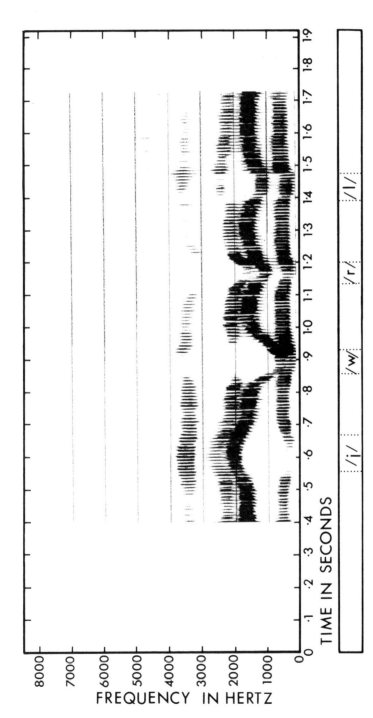

Figure 23. These are spectrograms of samples of the four vowellike consonants produced in the context of the vowel /ɛ/ (head). Note that the articulatory movements of the glides /w/ and /j/ are reflected in rapid changes of formant frequency. Note also the sudden changes of spectrum as the tongue touches and leaves the palate in the production of /l/.

lowered, thus opening the velopharyngeal port. Indeed, these are the only sound patterns of English that require the velum to be lowered. The mouth is closed at the lips, the alveolar ridge, or the soft palate, producing, respectively, the bilabial /m/ (*sum*), the alveolar /n/ (*sun*), or the velar /ŋ/ (*sung*).

The spectrograms of nasals are characterized by low amplitude and a predominance of low formants of fixed frequency. The differences between the three nasals are seen not so much in their own spectra as in the formant changes in the adjacent vowels as the articulators move to and from the nasal configuration. These changes are illustrated in Figure 24.

Fricatives

Fricatives come in two varieties, voiceless and voiced. For the voiceless fricatives the sole sound source is frication. For the voiced fricatives there are two sound sources, frication and voicing. For both types of consonant the sole resonator is the oral cavity. The shape of this cavity (and therefore the frequencies of the formants) is largely determined by the place at which frication is produced. In English there are six voiceless fricatives, distinguished from each other according to the location of the sound source (see Figure 25):

1. /ʍ/ (*whence*) uses, as its sound source, frication produced by turbulent air flow between the lips (bilabial). The frication is of very low amplitude, partly because it is difficult to produce turbulent air flow between the lips and partly because there are, in front of the source, no cavities in which resonance can occur. The main acoustical properties of /ʍ/ are the absence of voicing and the rapid formant changes in the subsequent vowel as the lips move away from the almost closed position. If we add voicing to /ʍ/, the reduction of air flow caused by the periodic vibration of the vocal cords eliminates the frication altogether, and we are left with the vowellike consonant /w/. In fact, most speakers omit the /ʍ/ sound from their consonant system and use /w/ instead.

2. /f/ (*fin*) uses, as its sound source, frication produced by turbulent air flow between the lower lip and the upper teeth (labiodental). The frication is of low amplitude, partly because it is difficult for air to flow between the teeth and partly because there is, in front of the source, little space in which resonance can occur. Such resonance as does occur tends to be very high in frequency.

3. /θ/ (*thin*) uses, as its sound source, frication produced by turbulent air flow between the tongue and the upper teeth (linguadental). Acoustically /θ/ is very similar to /f/; indeed, the two are easily confused. The major differences between the two are likely to be seen (and heard) in the changes of

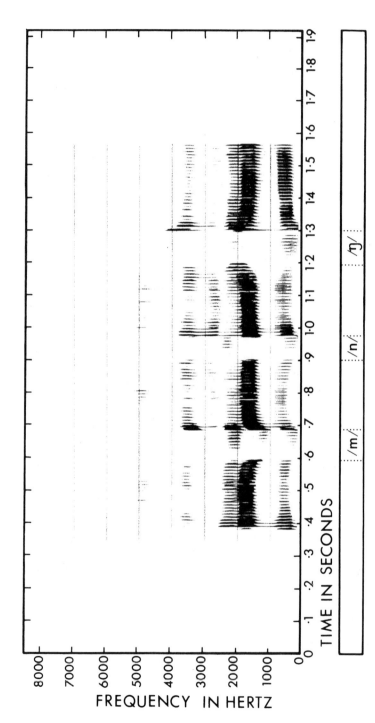

Figure 24. The three nasal consonants use the nasal cavity as the sole resonator. All three have similar spectra and a low amplitude. The differences are observed in the changes of formant frequency in the adjacent vowel as the articulators move to and from the positions required by the nasals.

formant frequency in neighboring sounds as the articulators move to and from their respective positions.

4. /s/ (*sin*) uses, as its sound source, frication produced by turbulent air flow between the tongue and the alveolar ridge (alveolar). The /s/ sound is of high amplitude, partly because the space in which turbulence occurs is relatively long and partly because there is a resonant cavity in front of the source. The resonant frequencies are high, typically above 4000 Hz, and the spectrum of /s/ therefore consists mainly of high frequencies.

5. /ʃ/ (*shin*) uses, as its sound source, frication produced by turbulent air flow between the tongue and the hard palate (palatal). Like /s/, this is a high-amplitude sound. Its spectrum, however, contains lower frequencies than /s/ because of resonance in the 2000 to 4000 Hz range. Because they are of high amplitude, the sounds /s/ and /ʃ/ are referred to as *sibilants*.

6. /h/ (*hid*) uses, as its sound source, frication produced between partially closed vocal cords (glottal). The spectrum of /h/ is that of a random noise with the formant structure of the subsequent vowel. The /h/ sound is also referred to as the *aspirate*.

The voiced fricatives are the first type of speech sound we have considered in which there are two sound sources. Voiced fricatives are produced by bringing the vocal cords together so that the air is released in periodic bursts and then allowing this air to produce turbulence by creating a narrow space through which it must pass. Three of the fricatives just described do not have voiced counterparts. It has already been pointed out that the addition of voicing to /ʍ/ produced the vowellike consonant /w/. Similarly, the addition of voicing to /h/ produces a vowel. This leaves four voiced fricatives (see Figure 26):

1. /v/ (*van*), produced by adding voicing to /f/

2. /ð/ (*these*), produced by adding voicing to /θ/

3. /z/ (*zoo*), produced by adding voicing to /s/

4. /ʒ/ (*pleasure*), produced by adding voicing to /ʃ/

The addition of voicing to a fricative has two main acoustical effects. First there is the addition of periodicity to an otherwise random noise. The result is neither a random noise nor a complex tone, but a mixture of the two. The second effect is a reduction in the amplitude of the frication. This occurs because the amplitude of frication is directly dependent on the rate of air flow, and this rate is reduced when the vocal cords come together and release the air in periodic bursts. These effects can be seen in the spectrograms of Figures 25 and 26.

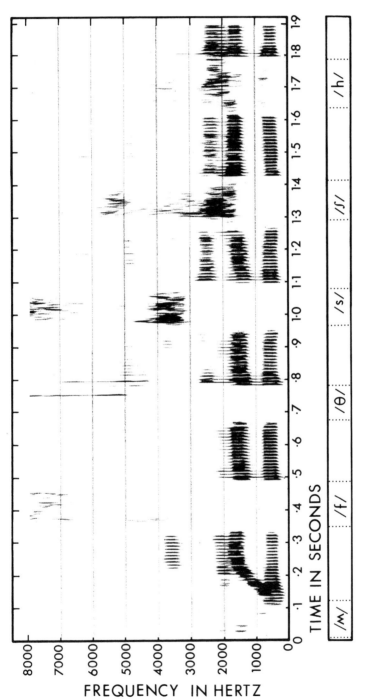

Figure 25. These are spectrograms of six voiceless fricatives produced in the context of the vowel /ɛ/ *(head)*. Note that they all consist of random noise but with different amplitudes and spectra, depending on the place of articulation. The /ʍ/ is a voiceless version of /w/; /f/ and /θ/ are very weak, and any resonances that occur are in the very high frequencies; /s/ and /ʃ/ are of relatively high amplitude but with energy concentrations in different frequency regions; the /h/ is like a voiceless version of the vowel that follows.

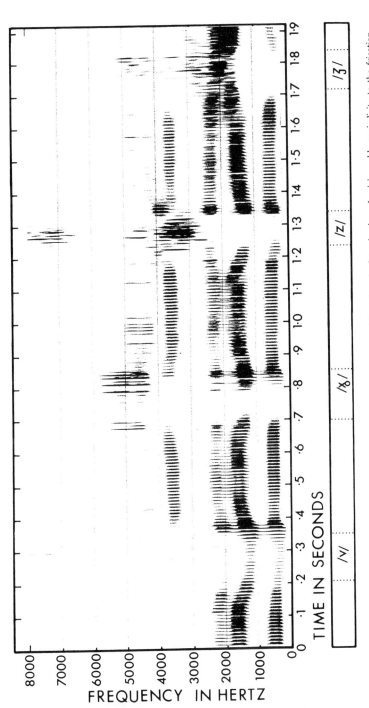

Figure 26. Four of the voiceless fricatives have voiced counterparts. Note that the introduction of voicing adds periodicity to the frication but reduces its amplitude.

The exact way in which voicing is added to frication is partly dependent on context. When the fricative occurs after a vowel, for example, the presence of voicing may be signaled by adding duration to the vowel. Sometimes this is the only cue to voicing, the fricative portion itself being produced without voicing. Consider, for example, the word *eyes*. Phonemically, the final sound is a /z/, but acoustically it is an *s* preceded by an elongated vowel. This is illustrated in Figure 27, in which spectrograms of the words *eyes* and *ice* are contrasted.

Stop-Plosives

Like the fricatives, *stop-plosives* come in two varieties, voiceless and voiced. For the voiceless variety the sole sound source is voicing. For the voiced variety there are two sound sources, stop-plosion and voicing. The sole resonator is the oral cavity, its shape being largely determined by the place at which stop-plosion is produced. There are three voiceless stop-plosives (see Figure 28):

1. /p/ (*pin*) is produced by blocking the air flow at the lips (bilabial). The burst of frication that occurs when the built-up air pressure is released is of relatively low amplitude. Its spectrum is similar to that of /ʍ/.

2. /t/ (*tin*) is produced by blocking the air flow with the tongue and the alveolar ridge (alveolar). The burst of frication that occurs when the built-up pressure is released is of relatively high amplitude. Its spectrum is similar to that of /s/.

3. /k/ (*kin*) is produced by blocking the air flow with the tongue and either the hard or the soft palate (palatal or velar). The burst of frication that occurs when the built-up pressure is released is of relatively high amplitude.

Voiced stop-plosives are produced by adding voicing during the production of stop-plosion. The voicing may be added during the closure, in which case the rate at which air flows into the blocked oral cavity is reduced. This reduces the rate at which pressure builds up behind the blockage, which, in turn, reduces the strength of the plosive burst when the blockage is released. Alternatively, voicing may begin immediately after the release of the blockage. In either case, there is a reduction in the rate of air flow during the production of the fricative portion and a consequent reduction in the amplitude of the brief burst of frication. Each of the three voiceless stop-plosives has a voiced counterpart (see Figure 29):

1. /b/ (*bin*) is produced by adding voicing to /p/.
2. /d/ (*din*) is produced by adding voicing to /t/.
3. /g/ (*gun*) is produced by adding voicing to /k/.

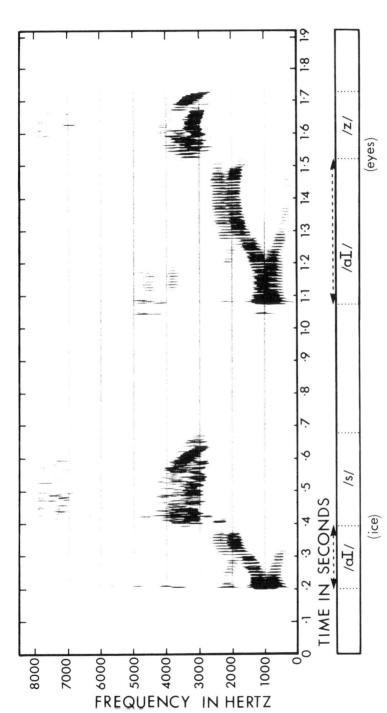

Figure 27. Voicing of a word-final fricative is revealed as a prolongation of the previous vowel rather than as the addition of voicing to the frication, as illustrated in these spectrograms of the words *ice* (/aɪs/) and *eyes* (/aɪz/).

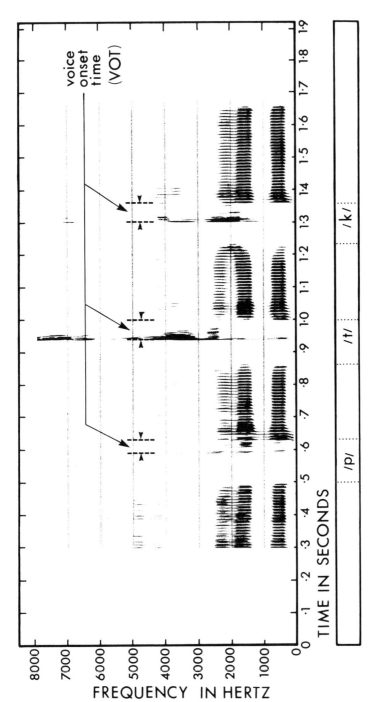

Figure 28. These are spectrograms of samples of the three voiceless stop-plosives in the context of the vowel /ɛ/ (*head*). Note how each shows a period of silence during the stop, the sudden appearance of random noise as the stop is released, and the appearance of formants during a brief period of frication. The voice onset time (VOT) is the interval between the release of the stop and the appearance of voicing for the following vowel. In these samples, the VOT is about 1/20th of a second. This is long enough to permit completion of the fricative burst.

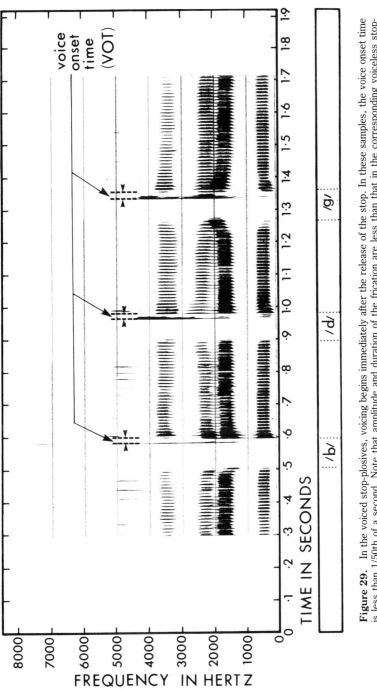

Figure 29. In the voiced stop-plosives, voicing begins immediately after the release of the stop. In these samples, the voice onset time is less than 1/50th of a second. Note that amplitude and duration of the frication are less than that in the corresponding voiceless stop-plosives.

It will be seen from Figures 28 and 29 that the main acoustical features of a stop-plosive are as follows: a period of silence (or of very low-intensive, low-frequency voiced sound if there is voicing into a closed oral cavity); the sudden appearance of energy across a wide range of frequencies; and a brief period of frication with clear evidence of formant structure and a rapidly decreasing amplitude.

In context, some of these features may be missing. For example, if the stop-plosive is the first sound in an utterance, the silent period will not be evident since there is no prior sound with which to contrast it. If the stop-plosive is the last sound in an utterance, the speaker has the option not to release the built-up pressure, in which case there will be no sudden onset of noise and no fricative burst. These effects are illustrated in Figure 30.

The acoustical features introduced by voicing also depend on the context within which the stop-plosive is produced. In a voiceless stop-plosive that occurs at the beginning of an utterance, there is a delay of at least 1/20th of a second between the release of the built-up pressure and the onset of voicing for any vowel that follows. This time, which is known as the *voice onset time* (VOT), is sufficient to allow the burst of fricative noise to be completed without interference from the voicing. When the same stop-plosive is voiced, the voicing is either present at the moment of release of the built-up pressure or begins within about 1/50th of a second (i.e., the VOT is much shorter). These differences can be seen in the spectrograms of Figures 28 and 29.

When a voiced stop-plosive is produced at the end of an utterance, the presence of voicing may be signaled by increasing the duration of the preceding vowel and by extending the voicing into the otherwise silent period (see Figure 31).

Affricates

There are two *affricates* in English, one voiceless and one voiced. Sample spectrograms are shown in Figure 32. The voiceless affricate has two sound sources, frication and stop-plosion. Essentially it is the fricative /ʃ/ with a plosive onset. The sole resonator is the oral cavity. The two affricates are as follows:

1. /tʃ/(*chair*) is produced by blocking air flow with the tongue just behind the alveolar ridge, releasing the built-up pressure, and then holding the tongue close to the palate long enough to produce an extended period of frication.

2. /dʒ/(*jar*) is produced by adding voicing to /ʒ/. It is the only speech sound pattern in English that uses all three types of sound source.

The articulatory classification of consonants just presented is summarized in Table 2.

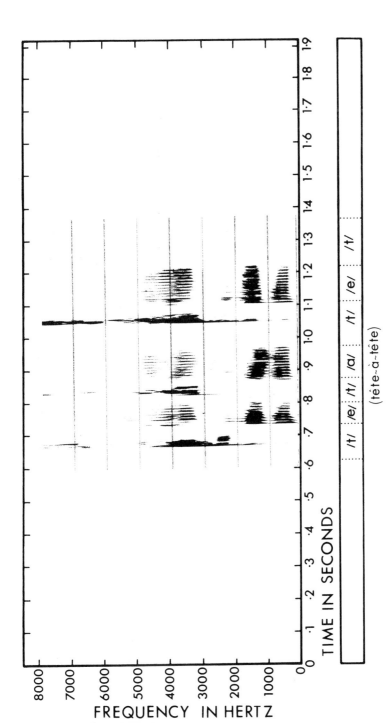

Figure 30. This spectrogram of *tête-a-tête* shows that the silence during an initial stop-plosive cannot be distinguished from the silence that preceded it and that the plosive portion may be omitted from a final stop-plosive. This example illustrates the influence of phonetic context on the patterns of speech movement (and therefore speech sound) that may be used to represent a given phoneme.

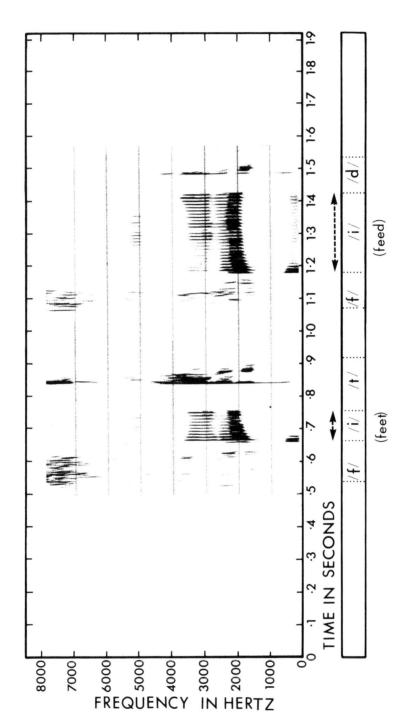

Figure 31. As with fricatives, the voicing of a final stop-plosive may be revealed by lengthening the preceding vowel rather than by adding voicing during the closure and release. This is illustrated in these spectrograms of the words *feet* and *feed*.

TABLE 2
Classification of English Consonants by Place of Articulation, Presence or Absence of Voicing, and Type (or Manner of Articulation)

Place of Articulation	Presence or Absence of Voice	Consonant Type				
		Vowel-like	Nasal	Fricative	Stop-Plosive	Affricate
Bilabial	Voiceless			/ʍ/	/p/	
	Voiced	/w/	/m/		/b/	
Labiodental	Voiceless			/f/		
	Voiced			/v/		
Linguadental	Voiceless			/θ/		
	Voiced			/ð/		
LinguaAlveolar	Voiceless			/s/	/t/	
	Voiced	/j/	/n/	/z/	/d/	
Linguapalatal	Voiceless			/ʃ/		/tʃ/
	Voiced	/r/ | /l/		/ʒ/		/dʒ/
Linguavelar	Voiceless				/k/	
	Voiced		/ŋ/		/g/	
Glottal	Voiceless			/h/		
	Voiced					

Features

A feature may be defined as a dimension along which changes of speech pattern are used to differentiate phonemic categories. Thus, the consonant system of English can be completely specified in terms of three features: *manner* of production (vowellike, nasal, fricative, stop-plosive, or affricate), *voicing* (voiced or voiceless), and *place* of articulation (with seven possibilities). There is, for example, only one alveolar, voiced, fricative (namely, /z/). This three-feature system for classifying consonants is commonly used by speech-language pathologists. Other feature systems have been developed, the best known being the "distinctive feature" system of Chomsky and Halle.

Syllables

When we examine the acoustic patterns of connected speech, we note that it consists of alternations between the longer, louder vowels and clusters of the

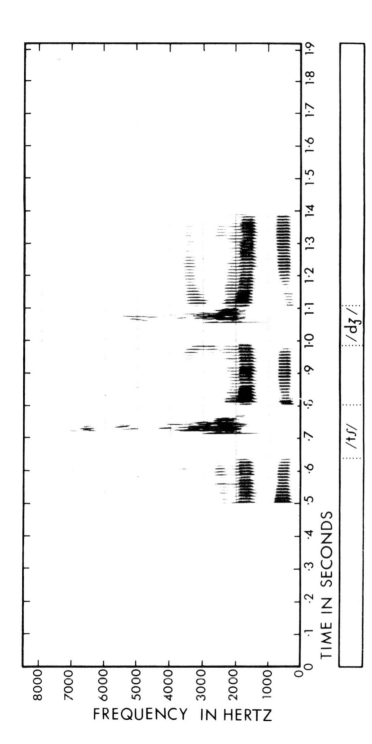

Figure 32. These are spectrograms of samples of the affricates /tʃ/ and /dʒ/ in the context of the vowel /ɛ/ (*head*). The affricates are essentially fricatives with a stop-plosive onset. Note that the VOTs are considerably longer than those for stop-plosives. Note also the difference in VOT between the voiced and voiceless affricate as well as the reduction of frication amplitude with voicing.

shorter, weaker consonants. If we divide, or segment, the speech stream at the consonants, we produce small units called *syllables*. A single syllable consists of a vowel nucleus that begins and ends with anywhere from zero to three consonants. The word *eye*, for example, consists of a single syllable with a vowel nucleus (V) and no consonants at beginning and end. The word *tie* consists of a single syllable with a vowel nucleus and one consonant at the beginning (CV). Similarly, the word *eyed* is a VC syllable, the word *hide* is a CVC syllable, the word *stripes* is a CCCVCC syllable, and so on.

Coarticulation

Just because we can represent connected speech by streams of discrete phonetic symbols, it should not be assumed that real speech is produced as a sequence of separate and distinct movement patterns. On the contrary, when we examine connected speech we find that the various sections of the speech mechanism move continuously, producing continuous changes in the resulting acoustical patterns. A perfect example of this phenomenon can be found in Figure 13. In effect, the movement patterns representing consecutive phonemes overlap so that, at any instant in time, the configuration of the speech mechanism is the result of the combined effects of two or even more phonemes. The term *coarticulation* is used to refer to the process of overlapping and combining the movement patterns required for sequentially produced phonemes.

The process of coarticulation makes itself apparent in the spectograms of connected speech where the acoustical patterns of a given sound are modified by what comes before and after. Just as the movement patterns for adjacent phonemes overlap, so do the resulting acoustical patterns.

Coarticulation can take several forms. When we produce a particular sound pattern, there are often articulators whose position is of little or no immediate importance. The articulators will usually be moved into position in anticipation of the next sound. Consider, for example, the word *team*. The velum needs to be raised for the production of /t/ but will be lowered for the production of /m/. Although it is usual to produce the /i/ with a raised velum, it makes more sense in this context to lower the velum during the /i/ so that it will already be in the lowered position when the lips are brought together for the /m/. In this way we coarticulate the /i/ and the /m/. Similarly, in the word *play*, the position of the tongue is irrelevant to the production of /p/, providing it does not block the oral cavity. We therefore usually move the tongue into the /l/ position during the stop portion of the /p/, thereby coarticulating the /p/ and the /l/.

Another manifestation of coarticulation is a change of lip configuration during consonant production in anticipation of a subsequent vowel. If you stand in front of a mirror and say *seesaw*, for example, you will see that the lip configurations for the two versions of /s/ anticipate the configurations needed for the vowels. The differences of configuration produce corresponding differences of acoustical properties.

When the same articulator is needed for the production of two sounds in sequence, we often change the place of articulation for the first sound so as to simplify the transition to the next sound. Consider, for example, the words *keel* and *cool*. In anticipation of the tongue positions required for the vowels we typically produce the first /k/ as far forward as we can, usually against the hard palate, but we produce the second /k/ as far back as we can, usually against the soft palate.

On a spectrogram, the effects of coarticulation may be seen either as a change of spectrum with changing phonetic context, or as a rapid change of formant frequencies as the articulators move between sound positions.

Suprasegmentals

So far we have considered only those sound patterns that are combined sequentially to produce words. These are referred to as the *segments* of speech. When we produce words, phrases, and sentences, there are aspects of the resulting patterns that stretch across many segments. These are known as *suprasegmental* features. We shall consider two of them, intonation and rhythm.

Intonation

Intonation is the name we give to the patterns of variation of fundamental frequency over time. Intonation is carried by the voiced sounds of speech (i.e., the vowels, vowellike consonants, and the nasals). There is much that we do not know about the way we plan and implement the intonation patterns of speech. A few points have, however, been established.

The basic intonation pattern of an English sentence consists of a constant or slowly falling fundamental frequency with a rapid fall at the end. This "terminal fall" is produced by a reduction of subglottal pressure and vocal cord tension.

When we pause in the middle of a sentence, either to take a breath, to collect our thoughts, or for special effect, we omit the terminal fall, thus indicating to the listener that our thought is not finished. If we wish to leave the

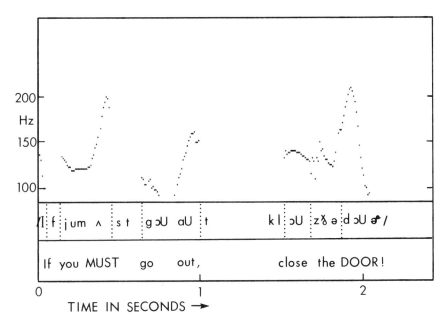

Figure 33. The basic English sentence has a constant or steadily falling fundamental frequency with a marked fall of fundamental frequency at the end. Nonterminal pauses are marked by the absence of a fall, or possibly a rise of fundamental frequency. Stress and emphasis are conveyed by a change of fundamental frequency from the general contour. This change is usually a rise but can also be a drop.

listener in no doubt about our intention to continue, we may introduce a rise of fundamental frequency before the pause. This same technique can be used when we wish to pressure the listener into completing the thought, either by answering a question (e.g., "Has it stopped raining yet?") or by confirming or denying the truth of a statement (e.g., "That's yours?").

During a sentence we use changes of fundamental frequency to add stress or emphasis to a syllable or word. The change is usually a rise but can be a fall. Its purpose is to bring the listener's attention to bear on an important word or syllable. The intonation contour of a typical sentence is shown is Figure 33.

Rhythm

Rhythm refers to the timing patterns of speech. It is determined by the relative durations of the sounds and syllables, by the relative time intervals between stressed syllables, and by the position and durations of pauses. As with inton-

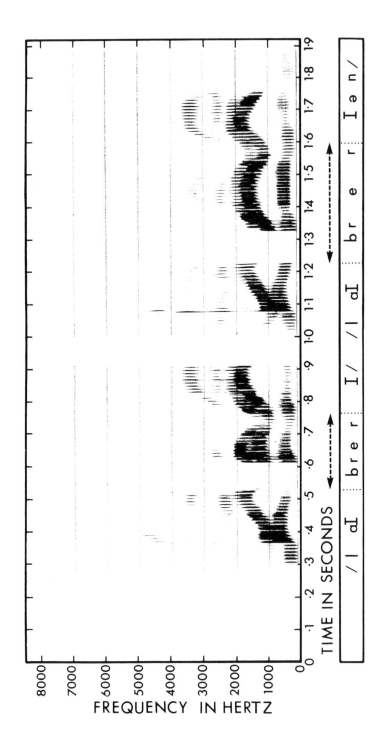

Figure 34. Stressed syllables are marked by an increase of duration, as shown in these spectrograms of utterances of *library* and *librarian*. The second syllable (/brɛr/) lasts roughly 250 thousandths of a second in the former and 350 thousandths in the latter.

ation, we are a long way from understanding the underlying rules governing the rhythm of speech. Nevertheless, a few points have been established.

Stressed syllables are typically increased in duration while unstressed syllables are reduced in duration. Thus the same syllable may change in duration by a factor of two or more if it shifts from a stressed position to an unstressed position. This is seen in the spectrogram of Figure 34, where the second syllable (/brɛr/) is twice as long in *librarian* as it is in *library*.

When a stressed syllable occurs just before the end of a sentence, it is made extra long, and if a pause must be introduced in a sentence, it is more likely to occur between phrases rather than within them. Thus pauses and syllable lengthening may assist the listener is determining the syntactic structure of connected speech.

PART FOUR

The Sense of Hearing

Animals depend for survival on their ability to acquire information about the environment (see Figure 35). To this end they have developed several sensory systems, the best known being those of vision, hearing, touch, taste, and smell. Each sensory system consists of two parts. The first is a sense organ in which physical stimuli from the environment are converted into patterns of nerve stimulation. The second is a set of specially developed brain structures that interpret the patterns of nerve stimulation. In the case of hearing, the sense organ consists of the outer, middle, and inner ears, and the brain structures are the auditory pathways and auditory processing centers. It is important to realize that most of what we call "hearing" takes place not in the ear but in the brain. The ear's task is to collect sound energy, to convey it to the fluids of the inner ear, and to transform the patterns of fluid movement into patterns of electrical stimulation in the auditory nerve. It is in the brain that these patterns give rise to the sensation of hearing, and it is in the brain that they are interpreted.

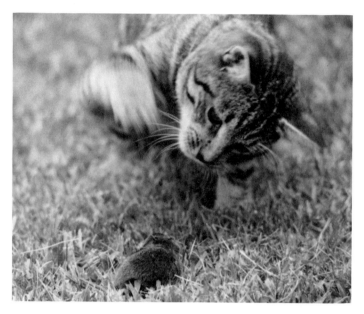

Figure 35. Animals require information about the world around them if they are to find their way around, locate mates, find food, avoid predators, etc. To this end they have developed sensory systems for the detection and interpretation of physical stimuli produced by the substances, objects, and events that constitute the environment.

Perception

Perception is the name we give to the reception and interpretation of physical stimuli via our sensory systems. The process involves several components (see Figure 36):

1. *Distal stimulus*. First there is the substance, object, or event that is to be perceived — for example: cheese, a chair, or a falling rock. Some writers call this the distal stimulus because it is remote from us. Even when we are touching an object, we do not have direct access to what we are perceiving, but only to physical evidence such as pressure and temperature.

2. *Proximal stimulus*. Perception is only possible because the distal stimulus produces physical evidence of itself. Examples are molecules released into the surrounding air, patterns of light reflected from its surface, or in the case of an event, disturbances of the air (i.e., sound waves). It is this evidence that provides the physical stimulus for the sense organ. To distin-

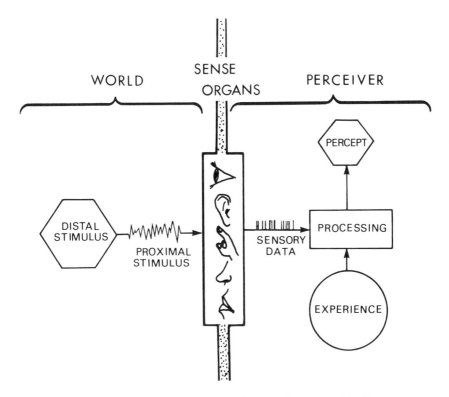

Figure 36. Perception involves the interpretation of sensory data generated by the sense organs in response to stimuli that originate from the object or event being perceived. The resulting internal representation of the object or event is known as the percept.

guish the physical stimulus from its cause, some writers refer to this stimulus as the proximal stimulus, thus emphasizing its direct impact on the sense organ.

3. *Sensory data*. The proximal stimulus causes the sense organ to generate patterns of electrical stimulation in nerve fibers connected to the brain. These patterns constitute the sensory data, or sensory evidence, on which the brain will base decisions about the nature of the proximal and distal stimuli.

4. *Processing*. Interpretation of sensory data is often referred to as sensory processing.

5. *Percept.* The result of processing is a percept. This may be thought of as an internal representation of the distal stimulus. In this way we smell "cheese," we see "a chair," and we hear "a rock falling."

Auditory Perception

When we refer to *auditory perception* we are speaking of perception via the sense of hearing. In this case, the distal stimulus is an event, the proximal stimulus is sound, the sense organ is the ear, the sensory data consist of patterns of electrical stimulation in the auditory nerve, processing is the operation that takes place in the auditory centers of the brain, and the resulting percept is an internal representation of the original event.

The details of how we accomplish auditory perception are not well understood. We can, however, identify some of its components. These will be discussed in turn.

Detection

Detection of a sound occurs when at least one of its component pure tones falls within the frequency range of hearing (20 Hz to 20,000 Hz) and has sufficient amplitude to have a significant effect on the patterns of electrical stimulation in the auditory nerve. If all other sound sources have been removed, then this amplitude is known as the *threshold of hearing*. The threshold of hearing varies with frequency, but over the most sensitive region, that is, 500 Hz to 4000 Hz, we can detect sounds in which the pressure of the air in the ear canal fluctuates by only about 10 billionths of its steady value. In hearing test equipment, the amplitude of sound at the threshold of hearing is assigned a value of 0 dB.

Sound Sensation

Stimulation of the sense of hearing produces a sensation that is different from the sensations produced by stimulation of the eye or the skin. We refer to this sensation as *sound*, a term also used to refer to the physical stimulus to which the ear responds. This use of a single term to describe two different things can be confusing and has led to futile arguments about whether a sound can exist in the absence of a listener. You can avoid confusion if you use the term *sound stimulus* for the patterns of movement in the air and the term *sound sensation* for the sensation produced when those patterns stimulate the sense of hearing.

The sound sensation has many dimensions, each of which is related to a dimension of the sound stimulus. The three principal dimensions of sound sensation are as follows:

1. *loudness*, which depends primarily on the amplitude of the sound stimulus, with equal decibel increases of amplitude producing roughly equal increases of loudness;

2. *pitch*, which depends primarily on the frequency (or, in the case of complex tones, the fundamental frequency) of the sound stimulus, with equal multiplication of frequency producing roughly equal increases of perceived pitch;

3. *quality* (i.e., that which distinguishes the sounds of a violin, a flute, and a piano when they are playing the same note), which depends on both the spectrum and the time/intensity envelope of the sound stimulus.

Discrimination

If we are to gain information about events occurring in the environment, it is not sufficient that the organ of hearing simply detect a sound stimulus and that the brain experience a sound sensation. The information carried by sound resides in the differences among sound stimuli. The hearing system must therefore be capable of responding to those differences by producing different sensations. The process of detecting differences between sound stimulus patterns is referred to as *discrimination*.

Experiments have shown that the sense of hearing is remarkably sensitive to differences of frequency. Over most of the frequency range we can detect frequency changes of about 1% (a musical step of one semitone, the difference between a white note and an adjacent black note on a piano, represents a frequency change of about 6%). This ability to detect small frequency changes gives us about 1,000 discriminable steps between 20 Hz and 20,000 Hz.

Our sensitivity to changes of amplitude is less acute. Here we require a change of about 10%, which translates into about 1 dB. This gives us approximately 100 discriminable steps of amplitude between the threshold of hearing and the level at which sound becomes uncomfortably loud.

We have good discrimination ability in the dimension of time. We can detect differences of about 10 millionths of a second in the timing of events at the right and left ears. With a single ear we can detect changes of quality resulting from time changes of about 1/1000th of a second, we can detect a brief interruption in sound of the order of a few thousandths of a second, and we can perceive the order of two events if they are separated by only 1/50th of a second.

Our ability to detect changes in the spectrum of a complex sound is also very good, due mainly to our excellent discrimination ability for frequency.

Localization

When we use hearing to learn about events occurring in the environment, it is important for us to find out not only what the events are but also where they have occurred. The ability to do this is known as *localization*. It is one of the first abilities developed by young children and may be capitalized on for assessment of hearing in infants. Information about the location of a sound source is obtained in a variety of ways. The most important is through differences in the sound patterns picked up by the right and left ears. These patterns differ both in timing, because of the finite speed of sound, and spectrum, because low frequencies travel around corners better than do high frequencies.

Recognition

Recognition refers to the correct identification of sensory data in terms of previously acquired knowledge. Recognition of a sound pattern occurs when we have identified its source – that is, when we have decided what the event was that caused the sound. In order to do this we must have learned from experience which features of the sound pattern are reliably associated with a particular type of event and which are likely to vary in an unpredictable manner. We can equate the end result of recognition with the percept which was discussed earlier.

It is important to realize that, when choosing a percept as the best possible interpretation of a given pattern of sensory data, our options, though numerous, are limited. As part of the process of perceptual development we organize our experience into a world model that has a finite number of object types, event types, and substance types. Similarly the attributes of objects, events, and substances (e.g., color, loudness, taste) become organized into a finite number of categories. The process of recognition is not therefore one of inventing a percept but of choosing among a set of preexisting, possible percepts. If we are not satisfied with any of the options, we may then find it necessary to invent a new percept or to refine an old one. In doing so, we are engaged not so much in perception as in perceptual development, a process that does not have to end with childhood.

Just how we decide which of numerous possible percepts best represents the source of a given pattern of sensory data is not well understood. The process is studied under the heading of *pattern recognition* and is currently of great interest to computer engineers who wish to improve the accuracy and speed or recognition of machines such as computers and robots, as well as to speech/language pathologists and learning disabilities specialists who are interested in the evaluation and remediation of persons with disorders of perception.

There are several ways of quantifying auditory recognition. The obvious technique is to record the proportion of occasions on which the percept corresponds with the distal stimulus. This provides an estimate of the probability of correct recognition. A second technique places the acoustic stimulus in a background of noise and determines the level of noise at which the probability of correct recognition is reduced to some predetermined value (typically 50%). A third approach is to record the time it takes for the subject to reach and indicate a perceptual decision. The first method provides a score in percentage, the second provides a signal-to-noise ratio in decibels, and the third provides a reaction time in milliseconds. By measuring these quantities and observing the ways in which they change in response to changes in the distal and proximal stimuli and their contexts, researchers are able to test hypotheses about the internal workings of the recognition process.

Comprehension

Auditory comprehension occurs when we correctly interpret a novel combination of recognized sound patterns. Whereas recognition results in the selection of one of many previously determined percepts, comprehension allows us to go beyond the limits of previous experience and to arrive at an interpretation that could have been predicted from our knowledge of the world but may never have been encountered before. If, for example, we walk past a car and hear sounds coming from inside the trunk, we may recognize them as coming from a human being who is in distress, but we must go beyond our previous experience if we are to comprehend that someone is trapped inside and wishes to get out. In colloquial terms, comprehension requires that we "put 2 and 2 together" in order to explain what has been recognized.

Attention

The processing centers of our brain are continually bombarded with information that our sense organs have generated from physical stimuli. If we are to function effectively, decisions must be made about which sensory data to deal with, how to monitor other sensory data, and when to shift priorities in the light of changing circumstances. The process of making and carrying out these decisions is referred to as *attentional behavior*.

Auditory attention involves such things as monitoring the acoustic input for important patterns, even though our primary attention may be to another modality such as vision; continuing to attend to an auditory input in the face of distractions from other modalities; and attending to one auditory signal in the face of competing auditory inputs. Some of the difficulties of auditory perception exhibited by brain-injured and developmentally delayed children can be attributed to deficiencies of attentional behavior.

Memory

If we are to process sensory data adequately, we must store and recall information. At least two kinds of memory are necessary. One is short-term memory, which allows us to hold on to one part of a stimulus pattern while waiting for the rest of the pattern to emerge, or to hold on to the whole pattern until we are ready to process it. The second is long-term memory, which permits us to benefit from all experiences and to use the resulting information to improve performance in the future. Both short-term memory and long-term memory are essential to auditory perception.

Auditory Perception as Questions and Answers

A useful way of thinking about perception is as the asking of questions about the environment and the answering of those questions on the basis of evidence provided by the sense organs. In the case of hearing, we ask questions about sounds and about the events that caused them. We answer those questions on the basis of evidence provided by our ears. The eight components of auditory perception just discussed can now be phrased in terms of questions and answers:

1. *detection*—asking and answering the question "Was there a sound?"

2. *sensation*—asking and answering the question "What was the sound like?"

3. *discrimination*—asking and answering the question "Did the sound change?" or "Was this sound different from that sound?"

4. *localization*—asking and answering the question "Where was the event that produced that sound?"

5. *recognition*—asking and answering the question "What was the event that caused the sound?"

6. *comprehension*—asking and answering the question "Why did that event occur?"

7. *attention*—deciding which questions to ask

8. *memory*—storing and recalling the answers

PART FIVE

Auditory Speech Perception

When we qualify the term *perception*, we may do so in terms both of what is being perceived and the sensory modality by which it is being perceived. Thus, speech perception is the perception of speech. Auditory speech perception is the perception of speech via the sense of hearing—that is, the reception and interpretation of the sound patterns of speech.

Note that it is also possible to perceive speech via the sense of vision, as with lipreading, and via the sense of touch, as with the Tadoma method used for communication with persons who are both deaf and blind. These processes may be referred to as visual speech perception and tactile speech perception, respectively. If two modalities are involved, as, for example, when a hard-of-hearing person both listens to and watches the facial movements of a speaker, we may indicate this with a double qualifier, as in auditory-visual speech perception. The following discussion is concerned with auditory speech perception, audition being the modality through which speech is intended to be perceived, and normally is.

The Distal Stimulus

You will recall that perception begins with a distal stimulus. One of the difficulties in any discussion of speech perception is the definition of the distal stimulus. The proximal stimulus is clearly the patterns of speech sound reaching our ear. These patterns carry evidence about the positions and movements of the speech mechanism, so it would appear at first sight that the distal stimulus consists of motor behaviors. These motor behaviors, however, are themselves evidence about phonemes. The phonemes, in turn, are evidence about words, and words occur in combinations called sentences that provide evidence of the meaning the speaker wishes to convey. Which, then, is the distal stimulus? Is it movements, phonemes, words, sentences, or meaning?

The only logical answer is "all of the above." The utterances of spoken language form a complex distal stimulus with many layers. At any given time a listener may be making perceptual decisions about an articulatory movement, about a phoneme, about a word, about the location of a syntactic boundary, about the location of a stress, or about the meaning of a sentence. There are even more layers to the distal stimulus. We may, for example, make decisions about the speaker's sex, country or region of origin, emotional state, and health. Although speech scientists have learned a lot about the acoustical cues that lead to specific perceptual decisions, there is still much we do not know about the strategies by which we arrive at an internal representation of this multilayered distal stimulus.

The issue of the distal stimulus can be simplified a little if we distinguish between recognition and comprehension. Essentially it is the phonemes and words that provide a finite set of possible percepts, and it is therefore appropriate to talk of phoneme and word recognition. We can also talk of the recognition of stress and syntactic boundaries. To the extent, however, that sentences and their meanings represent distal stimuli that are possible but have probably never been encountered before, it is more appropriate to refer to sentence perception under the heading of sentence comprehension. In the remainder of this section I shall focus on the recognition of phonemes, suprasegmental patterns, and words, these being the topics about which we have the most research data.

Phoneme Recognition

A considerable amount of research effort has been invested in discovering the acoustical features of speech sound patterns that are used for phoneme recognition. Two basically different approaches have been used. One involves removing acoustical details from real speech patterns and measuring the deterioration of recognition. The other involves the synthesis of artificial speech patterns and measuring the effects of adding or changing specific features of these patterns.

Early methods of speech synthesis used electrical sound generators and electrical filters to simulate the source-filter function of the speech mechanism. Current methods use computers to implement mathematical models of speech production and to calculate the acoustical waveforms. The following sections summarize the more important findings of this research.

Effects of Amplitude Change

If we start out with speech that is inaudible and gradually increase the amplitude, we reach a point at which the sound patterns are detectable but not recognizable. This may be referred to as the speech detection threshold. Speech is at detection threshold when the more intense sounds, typically the vowels /a/ and /ɔ/, are at the threshold of hearing. With a slight increase of amplitude, we are able to recognize a few phonemes, but an increase of about 30 dB is necessary before we can recognize all of them. The same range of 30 dB is found if we listen to speech in a background of noise and gradually increase the amplitude of the speech in relation to the noise. This phenomenon is easily explained. The weakest sounds, typically /f/ and /θ/, have an amplitude that is some 30 dB less than the strongest sounds, and we must therefore raise the strongest to 30 dB above detection threshold before the weakest become audible.

Effects of Filtering

The spectrum of speech includes frequencies as low as 70 Hz and as high as 10,000 Hz or even more, but not all frequencies in this range are equally important. During the early days of the commercial development of the telephone, a series of experiments was done to determine how much of the frequency range of speech could be sacrificed without having an undue effect on phoneme recognition. It was found that most (though not quite all) of the important acoustical information was contained in the range 300 to 3000 Hz. This is, in fact, the range of frequencies you now hear when communicating by telephone.

You will note that the range 300 to 3000 Hz is sufficient to include the frequencies of the first and second formants of the oral cavity. As we discuss the recognition of individual phonemes, it will become apparent that this is not mere coincidence.

Acoustical Cues to Sound Source

You will recall that the sound system of English uses three different sound sources. Voicing is recognized from the fact that the sound sensation has a tonal quality with a perceptible pitch. The acoustical features giving rise to tonicity are the periodicity of the waveform and the presence of a harmonic structure in the spectrum. It will be seen from many of the spectrograms discussed earlier that these cues are available across a broad frequency range, from perhaps 70 Hz to 4000 Hz, and are not limited, as is often assumed, to the very low frequencies. The fact that listeners can recognize the presence of voicing by using information from a broad range of frequencies has been confirmed in phoneme recognition experiments with filtered speech.

Frication is recognized from the fact that it produces a sound sensation with a "noisy," "hissing" quality. The acoustical features producing this quality are the randomness of the waveform and the absence of harmonic structure in the spectrum. Like the cues to voicing, these cues are also available across a broad range of frequencies. Since, however, many of the fricatives have the bulk of their spectral energy in the range above 2000 Hz, it is in this region that frication is most easily identified. The qualities of sensation associated with voicing and frication are not mutually exclusive. When both sources coexist, the cues to both are present and can be detected.

Stop-plosion is recognized from its characteristic time pattern – that is, a period of silence, or very low amplitude, followed by an almost instantaneous increase of amplitude. The spectrum of this sudden change of amplitude is like that of random noise and includes low, medium, and high frequencies. The presence of stop-plosion can, therefore, be determined from information contained in virtually any part of the frequency range of speech.

Vowel Recognition

That a phoneme is a vowel is determined from the fact that its sole sound source is voicing and that its spectrum has a clearly defined formant structure characteristic of oral resonance. Differentiation of short and long vowels is based partly on duration and partly on formant frequencies. Diphthongs as a class are identified from the formant changes resulting from movements of the tongue, jaw, and lips.

Within these categories, individual vowels are recognized from their formant frequencies, primarily the frequencies of F1 and F2. The process of vowel recognition, however, is not quite that simple. The average values of formant frequency change with vocal tract length, a parameter that is typically different for men, women, and children. Moreover, individual differences of anatomy and individual differences of speech posture, especially of the muscles of the pharyngeal walls, produce individual differences of average formant frequency independent of age and sex. Experiments have shown that these differences are accounted for by basing decisions not on absolute formant frequencies but on relative formant frequencies, particularly the ratio of the frequencies of F1 and F2.

The complications do not stop here. Vowel phoneme systems vary dramatically from country to country, and from region to region within a country, even when the same language is being spoken. That is to say, the typical oral cavity shape, and hence the pattern of formant frequencies, used for a given vowel phoneme may differ from region to region even though the resulting sounds play the same role in determining word meaning. It appears that we allow for these variations of dialect and other individual variations by adapting to the phoneme system of each speaker. The characteristics of this system are deduced, in part, by taking into account the possible meanings of the words and sentences we hear. This is one of many examples of the influence of word and sentence meaning on the recognition of speech at the phoneme level.

It will be seen from the foregoing that in order to identify individual vowels it is necessary to have access at least to that range of frequencies containing the first two oral cavity formants (i.e., roughly 300 to 3000 Hz). The cues that permit us to recognize vowels as a group and to distinguish among the three vowel types are also available in this frequency range.

Consonant Recognition

The vowellike consonants are recognized as a group from their voiced source and oral resonances. What makes them identifiably different from vowels are the rapid changes of formant frequency that accompany the movements of the articulators. Individual vowellike consonants are recognized from their formant frequencies, particularly at the moment of maximum closure of the oral cavity.

The nasals are recognized as a group from the fact that they have a voiced source, low amplitude, and a formant pattern characteristic of nasal resonance. Recognition of individual nasals is based not on the spectrum of the nasal sound itself but on the formant transitions in the adjacent vowels. These formant transitions provide the listener with information about the change in shape of the oral cavity just before and after the nasal and therefore indicate at which place oral closure was produced. Since the articulatory distinction among the three nasals is the place of blockage of the mouth in relation to the front and back, it is the frequency of the second vowel formant that provides the most useful cue as to which nasal is about to be produced, or was just produced.

Fricatives as a group are recognized from their fricative sound source. The fact that a fricative is voiced can be determined from several cues: the presence of low-frequency sound with a harmonic structure; the periodicity introduced into the fricative noise; the lowered amplitude of frication resulting from reduced air flow; or, in the case of word-final fricatives, the lengthening of the previous vowel.

Individual fricatives are identified primarily by the amplitude and spectrum of the fricative noise. You will recall that /s/ and /ʃ/ are of considerably higher amplitude than /h/, /f/, /θ/, or /ʍ/. The spectra and, in particular, the formant frequencies provide evidence about the shape of the oral cavity and therefore about the place at which frication was produced. Access to the important cues in the spectra of all fricatives would require access to a frequency range of perhaps 1000 Hz to 10,000 Hz or more. There are, however, additional clues to place of articulation in the formant transitions of adjacent vowels, as the articulators move to and from the position required for fricative production. Thus it may be sufficient to hear that a sound is a fricative and to identify its place of articulation from the second formant transition in the adjacent vowel in order to recognize it. This requires access only to the frequency range 900 to 3000 Hz.

The stop-plosives and affricates as a group are recognized primarily from their time envelope, in particular, from the sudden rise of amplitude at the moment of release of pressure in the oral cavity. The addition of voicing is recognized from several cues. When a vowel follows the consonant, both the short (or zero) voice onset time and the reduction of the amplitude of the burst of frication provide cues to voicing, and when a vowel precedes the consonant, the presence of voicing may be recognized from the increase in vowel duration. If a voiced stop-plosive or affricate is between two voiced sounds, the voicing typically continues during the stop and provides an additional cue to the listener.

The affricates are distinguishable from stop-plosives by the duration of the frication following the plosive release. Individual stop-plosives may be recognized either from the formants in the burst of frication or, like the fricatives, from the formant transitions in adjacent vowels. Once again, it is the frequency of the second formant that provides the most useful information about place of articulation of plosives. It is thus clear that there are situations in which more than one acoustical cue is available to the listener, any one being sufficient for recognition. The voicing of fricatives, for example, can be recognized either from the presence of voicing or from the reduction of frication amplitude. Similarly, the place of articulation of stop-plosives can be recognized either from the amplitude and spectrum of the burst of frication or from the formant transitions in the subsequent vowel. The simultaneous presence of two or more cues, each of which is sufficient for recognition, is known as *redundancy*, in this case, *acoustical redundancy*. The word *redundancy* does not, however, imply that something is unnecessary. Its presence protects the listener against loss of information, and when the multiple cues are used together, recognition usually occurs more quickly and with a lower probability of error.

Coarticulation

It was pointed out earlier that in connected speech the phonemes are not represented by separate, independent patterns of speech movement or speech sound. Rather, the movements and sound patterns of adjacent phonemes overlap. The result is that the sound pattern at any particular moment may represent the combined effects of several phonemes. How, then, can we recognize a phoneme if we cannot assume that it always results in the same sound pattern?

Considerable theoretical and research effort has been prompted by this question, and the answer is still not clear. One theory suggests that there are indeed invariant cues in some aspect of the acoustical pattern, or in some transform of the acoustical pattern. Another suggests that the acoustical patterns are first interpreted as movement patterns and that these are less variable. Even if there is not invariance at the motor level, the fact that the listener is also a producer of speech gives him or her special information about the constraints of the speech mechanism and the ways in which adjacent phonemes must interact.

Research has shown that listeners do modify their interpretations of acoustical patterns on the basis of phonemic context, presumably using prior information about the consequences of coarticulation. The appropriate interpretation of the findings of this research is, however, still a matter for discussion.

Recognition of Suprasegmentals

The main acoustical cues to the end of a sentence are an increase in duration of the last stressed syllable, a terminal fall of fundamental frequency, and the presence of a pause after the fall. If a pause is introduced in the middle of a sentence, either to mark a phrase boundary, to emphasize a word, or to give the speaker time to think of what to say next, the absence of a fall of fundamental frequency or the presence of a rise of fundamental frequency are cues to the fact that the sentence is not yet ended.

Stress is carried by three cues—duration, fundamental frequency change, and amplitude. Thus, a stressed word or syllable is made longer than it would otherwise be, its fundamental frequency is changed (usually upwards but sometimes downwards), and the amplitude is sometimes increased. Research has shown that a listener may use any one of these cues to identify stress, but that duration and fundamental frequency are more powerful cues than amplitude.

Word Recognition

It might be supposed that a word is recognized when its constituent phonemes have been recognized. Research has shown, however, that, under unfavorable listening conditions, the probability of recognition of a word is higher than that predicted from the combined probabilities of recognition of its phonemes. Moreover, the probability of word recognition is higher for common words than for uncommon words. One interpretation of this finding is that listeners identify a word as a complex acoustical pattern in its own right, without having first to identify each of its constituent phonemes.

It has also been shown that, under unfavorable listening conditions, words in sentence context are more easily recognized than words in isolation. This phenomenon appears to be due to the fact that, once the context of a word is defined, the number of possibilities for that word is reduced. Indeed, the phonemenon can be replicated by asking a listener to identify words that are selected from a closed set.

The three factors just mentioned, all of which increase the probability of recognizing a word under unfavorable listening conditions, have one characteristic in common. They increase the "a priori" probability for the words that are actually presented. Thus, whether we use common words rather than uncommon words, place words in sentence context, or give the listener a limited set from which the test word will be selected, we are increasing the listener's estimate of the probability of occurrence of the test word before he or she receives any acoustical cues. Note, however, that for the commonness of a word to have an effect on recognition, the listener must have had considerable experience with the vocabulary of that language. Similarly, for the sentence context to have an effect, the listener must have an intimate knowledge of syntax and of the things to which the sentences refer.

The fact that word familiarity, sentence context, sentence meaning, and situational context can have an effect on the probability of word recognition provides yet more examples of the redundancy in spoken language. In this case we have been discussing lexical, syntactic, semantic, and situational redundancy.

Theories of Speech Perception

Many theories have been developed to explain the processes by which a listener uses acoustical cues to arrive at decisions about articulatory movements, phoneme categories, words, stress, and syntactic boundaries. *Passive* theories suggest that the acoustical patterns of speech trigger phonemic and lexical responses when they match "templates" in the listener's brain. It is such theories that have prompted the search for acoustic invariance in the proximal stimulus mentioned earlier.

In contrast, *active* theories suggest that the listener makes hypotheses about the distal stimulus and then tests these hypotheses against the available evidence. This evidence consists both of the acoustical details in the proximal stimulus and the listener's knowledge of the situational context, the linguistic context, and the relationships among the many layers of the distal stimulus. Such theories do not require the existence of perfect invariants in the acoustical stimulus. Moreover, they provide a ready explanation for the general effects of acoustical and linguistic redundancy on phoneme and word recognition.

Theories of speech perception also differ in terms of the direction taken by the listener as he or she moves through the many layers of the distal stimulus. *Bottom-up* theories suggest that the listener first determines the phonemic content of the message, then uses this information as if it were the proximal stimulus for perception of the words. The words, together with information about syntactic structure and stress derived from the acoustical signal, serve as the raw material from which to reach decisions about sentences. Once the sentence structure has been defined, decisions can then be made about meaning.

In contrast, *top-down* theories suggest that the listener begins by trying to determine sentence meaning, descending to the sentence structure and content level only to resolve uncertainties about meaning. Similarly, the listener may descend to the word level to resolve uncertanties about sentence structure and content, and to the phoneme level if there are uncertainties about a particular word. The end result of a top-down and a bottom-up strategy would be the same—that is, perception of all layers of the distal stimulus. It is the method of reaching this end that would differ.

The *motor* theory of speech perception deals with the lowest layers of the distal stimulus—that is, the movement patterns and the resulting acoustical patterns. It is suggested that the first step in speech perception is the conversion of acoustical patterns into movement patterns and that the movement patterns then serve as the proximal stimulus for the rest of the speech perception process, regardless of whether it is active or passive, top-down or bottom-up. If this is so, then the search for acoustical invariance becomes a search for invariance in the movement patterns. In fact, the movement patterns of speech bear a more predictable relationship to the underlying phonemic structure than do the acoustical patterns. Moreover, each listener knows the relationship between movement patterns and acoustical patterns by virtue of being also a speaker.

At the time of writing there is much disagreement among speech and language scientists about the process involved in speech perception. A considerable body of data has been collected, but its interpretation often serves as a cause for further dispute rather than clarification. It is, of course, possible that the human listener is not constrained to a single speech perception strategy and that there is some truth in all existing theories. Alternatively a complete understanding of the process may have to await the development of some new theory. This is a fascinating and exciting field of study whose results have practical implications for such fields as computer recognition of speech, artificial intelligence, and the evaluation and treatment of spoken-language disorders.

Suggested Readings

Borden, G. J., & Harris, K. S. (1980). *Speech science primer*. Baltimore, MD: Williams & Wilkins.

Boothroyd, A. *Hearing impairments in young children*. Englewood Cliffs, NJ: Prentice-Hall, 1982.

Cairns, H. S. (1984). Research in language comprehension. In R. C. Naremore (Ed.), *Language science* (pp. 221–242). Austin, TX: PRO-ED.

Chomsky, N., & Halle, N. M. (1968). *The sound patterns of English*. New York: Harper & Row.

Davis, H., & Silverman, R. (1978). *Hearing and deafness*. New York: Holt, Rinehart, & Winston.

Denes, P., & Pinson, E. (1972). *The speech chain*. New York: Doubleday.

Droescher, V. B. (1971). *The magic of the senses*. New York: Harper & Row.

Durant, J. D., & Lovrinic, J. H. (1977). *Bases of hearing science*. Baltimore, MD: Williams & Wilkins.

Geldard, F. A. (1953). *The human senses*. New York: Wiley & Sons.

Gelfand, S. (1981). *Hearing: An introduction to psychological and physiological acoustics*. New York: Marcel Dekker.

Ladefoged, P. (1975). *A course in phonetics*. New York: Harcourt, Brace, Jovanovitch.

Lehiste, I. (1967). *Readings in acoustic phonetics*. Cambridge, MA: MIT Press.

Lieberman, P. (1977). *Speech physiology and acoustic phonetics: An introduction*. New York: Macmillan.

Minifie, F., Hixon, T. J., & Williams, F. (1972). *Normal aspects of speech, hearing, and language*. Englewood Cliffs, NJ: Prentice-Hall.

Pierce, J. R. (1984). *The science of musical sound*. New York: Scientific American Books.

Pickett, J. M. (1980). *The sounds of speech communication*. Austin, TX: PRO-ED.

Stevens, S. S. (1951). *The handbook of experimental psychology*. New York: Wiley & Sons.

Zemlin, W. R. (1968). *Speech and hearing sciences: Anatomy and physiology*. Englewood Cliffs, NJ: Prentice-Hall.

Arthur Boothroyd earned a B.S. degree in physics from the University of Hull in 1957 and a Ph.D. in audiology and deaf education from the University of Manchester in 1968. He was on the faculty of the University of Manchester from 1964 to 1968, at which time he moved to the United States to become Director of the Hudgins Diagnostic and Research Center at the Clarke School for the Deaf in Northampton, Massachusetts. Since 1981 he has been Professor of Speech and Hearing Sciences at the Graduate Center of the City University of New York. Dr. Boothroyd is well known for his research on the auditory capacities of severely and profoundly deaf children and on the use of sensory assistance devices in the management of speech perception and production difficulties in this population. He is the author of a text entitled *Hearing Impairments in Young Children.*